Local and Regional Flaps in Oral Cavity Cancer Reconstruction

Oral cavity cancer presents unique challenges due to the region's complex anatomy and vital functions. While microvascular reconstruction is the gold standard, it may not always be feasible due to limited resources, accessibility, advanced disease, or high post-operative care demands.

This practical color atlas draws on the authors' extensive experience to highlight local and regional flaps as effective alternatives in suitable cases. Featuring case examples, step-by-step guides, clear photographs, and access to operative videos, it provides a comprehensive yet accessible approach to reconstruction.

This color atlas serves as a valuable resource for both junior and senior colleagues in the field of oral cancer surgery. It offers a collection of cases to inspire alternative approaches when standard solutions may not suffice.

Surgical excellence lies in simplicity. While all authors are fully trained and practicing microvascular surgeons, the ability to achieve effective reconstruction with the appropriate technique is an art in itself.

Local and Regional Flaps in Oral Cavity Cancer Reconstruction

A Case-Based Approach

Muhammad Faisal
Abdul Ahmed
Raza Hussain
Michael Gilhooly

CRC Press
Taylor & Francis Group
Boca Raton London New York

CRC Press is an imprint of the
Taylor & Francis Group, an **informa** business

Designed cover image: Dr Catherine Lau

First edition published 2026
by CRC Press
2385 NW Executive Center Drive, Suite 320, Boca Raton, FL 33431

and by CRC Press
4 Park Square, Milton Park, Abingdon, Oxon, OX14 4RN

CRC Press is an imprint of Taylor & Francis Group, LLC

ISBN: 9781032714509 (hbk)
ISBN: 9781032714417 (pbk)
ISBN: 9781032714585 (ebk)

DOI: 10.1201/9781032714585

Typeset in Minion Pro
by KnowledgeWorks Global Ltd.

I would like to express my deepest gratitude to my mother, Shakeela, for shaping me into the person I am today; to my wife, Hania, for her unwavering and invaluable support, I cannot thank you enough for walking this journey with me; and to my children, Harrum and Abdullah, for filling my life with boundless joy and purpose. Being your parent is the greatest privilege I could ever have.

I am profoundly grateful to Dr. Arif Jamshed, Dr. Raza Hussain, and Professor Boban M. Erovic for being selfless mentors who have imparted to me the importance of compassion, resilience, and hard work.

I also extend my thanks to all the residents and fellows who have supported me over the years, offering their companionship and assistance.

Lastly, my heartfelt appreciation goes to all my patients, for without them, this book would not have been possible.

Muhammed Faisal

To my beloved wife, Shabana, and our wonderful children, Maryam and Raheem.

Shabana, your love, strength, and unwavering support make every journey worthwhile. Maryam and Raheem, your kindness, imagination, and boundless energy fill my heart with joy and remind me why I do what I do. You are my greatest inspiration and my proudest achievement.

This book is for you—may it always remind you that with passion, dedication, and belief in yourself, anything is possible.

Abdul Ahmed

Contents

Video List

Access to surgical videos demonstrating the surgical techniques for various flaps is available via the QR code.

Surgical Videos

Video 1 Neck Dissection

Video 2 Submental Flap

Video 3 Temporalis Flap

Video 4 Facial Artery Musculomucosal Flap (FAMM)

Video 5 Deltopectoral Flap

Video 6 Palatal Flap

Video 7 Pectoralis Major Flap

Video 8 Nasolabial Flap

Video 9 Buccal Fat Pad

Video 10 Platysma Flap

Video 11 Infrahyoid Flap

Foreword

It is a very great honor and pleasure for me to write the Foreword for the book *Local and Regional Flaps in Oral Cavity Cancer Reconstruction* by Muhammad Faisal, Abdul Ahmed, Raza Hussain, and Michael Gilhooly. It also fills me with great joy and makes me very proud to see that my former fellow, Dr. Muhammad Faisal, is one of the authors.

Every surgeon who is or has been involved in the surgical training of young doctors knows how difficult it is to create educational videos and images in such a way that they can fully develop their educational power. After reading the book and watching the videos, I am really impressed. The pictures alone are self-explanatory even for those young colleagues who have never seen or even performed the operations. The videos are of excellent quality, not only in terms of resolution quality but also in terms of the shooting angle. Since the camera's perspective corresponds to that of the surgeon, the educational power is particularly excellent.

The surgical performance in this book is exceptional; the techniques presented with monopolar and bipolar pick-and-flick cautery are perfect; and the surgical performance with HF surgical instruments is simply impressive. In addition to the perfect dissection techniques, many cases are presented and explained step by step.

I warmly recommend this book to all physicians who are or who are planning to work as head and neck surgeons. This book meticulously presents all relevant local and regional flaps needed for defect reconstruction in oral tumor surgery, not only to learn them but also to perfect them.

Professor Boban Erovic, MD
Vienna, Austria

Preface

ORAL CAVITY CANCERS PRESENT unique challenges due to the intricate anatomy and essential functions of this region. This requires optimal functional and aesthetic restoration involving complex reconstructive options for partial- or full-thickness defects.

With well-established microvascular reconstructive options, complex defects can be reconstructed to provide form and function as well as dental rehabilitation in complex anatomical environments. However, this is not always feasible and is practically impossible due to limited resources, high volume of advanced disease, patient factors, and complex post-operative care requiring specialized nursing and prohibitive costs.

According to GLOBOCON2020, oral cancer ranks among the most prominent cancers affecting males and stands as one of the top three prevalent cancers among females in Southeast Asia. The context of constrained financial resources and limited medical facilities places surgeons in a challenging position when considering advanced reconstructive procedures for patients. These procedures may appear more like extravagant choices than essential standards of medical care.

Within our medical facility, we attend to over 500 cases of head and neck cancer annually. This high caseload necessitates us to explore local and regional flap options as viable alternatives to the more intricate free flap reconstructions.

This book is a culmination of the collective knowledge drawn from the practical journeys of the authors in the realm of head and neck reconstruction, specifically employing local and regional flaps.

Dr. Muhammad Faisal
Professor Abdul Ahmed
Dr. Raza Hussain
Mr. Michael Gilhooly

Acknowledgements

THE AUTHORS EXTEND THEIR sincere gratitude to all the surgeons whose expertise, dedication, and invaluable contributions were instrumental in compiling this case series. Additionally, we are deeply appreciative of the patients who generously participated, allowing us to document and share these important clinical insights.

- *Dr. Ahmk Abeysinghe, Consultant, OMFS, National Hospital, Kandy, Sri Lanka*
- *Dr. Dayanath Kumara D. Dias, Consultant OMFS, National Hospital, Galle, Sri Lanka*
- *Mr. Michael Amin, Consultant OMFS, Wexham Park Hospital, UK*
- *Mr. Mahesh Kumar, Consultant OMFS, Hillingdon Hospital, London, UK*
- *Mr. Axel Martin, Consultant Head and Neck, University College London, UK*
- *Dr. Muhammad Umar Qayyum, Consultant Head and Neck Surgeon, Combined Military Hospital, Gujranwala, Pakistan*
- *Dr. Romana Mir, Consultant Clinical Oncologist, Mount Vernon Cancer Centre, London, UK*
- *Dr. Muhammad Mizanur Rahman, Consultant OMFS, Bangladesh*
- *Dr. Md. Mostafizur Rahman, Consultant OMFS, Shaheed Suhrawardy Medical College Hospital, Dhaka, Bangladesh*
- *Dr. Mostafij Rahman, Consultant OMFS, Bangladesh*
- *Mr. Keval Shah, Consultant OMFS, Northwick Park Hospital, London, UK*

- *Dr. Rahim Ullah Chowdhury, Consultant OMFS, Bangladesh*
- *Ms. Radhika Dua, Head and Neck Fellow, Northwick Park Hospital, UK*
- *Dr. Uzair Luqman, Consultant OMFS, Islamic International Dental College, Islamabad, Pakistan*
- *Dr. Arif Jamshed, Clinical Oncologist, Shaukat Khanum Memorial Cancer Hospital and Research Centre, Lahore, Pakistan*

Authors

Dr. Muhammad Faisal, BDS, FCPS (OMFS), FDSRCS, FHNS is a

- *Consultant, Oral and Maxillofacial/Head and Neck and Reconstructive Surgeon*
- Shaukat Khanum Memorial Cancer Hospital and Research Centre, Lahore, Pakistan
- International Clinical Supervisor, Head and Neck Oncology, EACMFS, Lahore, Pakistan
- Co-Director, Head and Neck Fellowship Program, SKMCH&RC, Lahore, Pakistan

Dr. Muhammad Faisal's surgical expertise, coupled with a strong passion for cancer research, has earned him recognition among his peers. His research focuses on identifying factors that influence treatment outcomes for head and neck cancers, leading to valuable insights and collaborations in multi-center studies. His unwavering commitment to both clinical excellence and scientific advancement continues to drive progress in cancer care.

Professor Abdul Ahmed, BDS, MFDSRCS, MBChB, MRCS, DO-HNS, PGCert, FRCS(OMFS)

- *Consultant, Oral and Maxillofacial/Head and Neck/Reconstructive Surgeon*
- London Northwest University NHS Trust, London, United Kingdom
- Professor (Hons), Oral and Maxillofacial Surgery, BAM&DC, Multan
- Honorary Senior Clinical Lecturer, Queen Mary University of London
- Honorary Clinical Lecturer, University College London

Professor Ahmed has over a decade of experience as a Consultant in OMFS and Head and Neck Surgery, he adopts an innovative approach to his practice, integrating cutting-edge technologies such as 3D planning, augmented reality, and robotic surgery.

A prolific author, Professor Ahmed has written multiple textbooks on maxillofacial surgery, microvascular surgery, and head and neck cancer. His commitment to education extends to teaching engagements at various universities, where he leads courses in microvascular surgery, reconstructive surgery, and undergraduate/postgraduate training. Additionally, he is a national and international speaker, delivering lectures and conducting specialized courses worldwide.

Professor Ahmed also plays a key role in surgical education and governance. He serves as the Regional Specialty Advisor for the Royal College of Surgeons and as an Educational Supervisor for the London School of Surgery.

Dr. Raza Hussain, MBBS, BDS, FDSCRCS, FFDRCSI

- *Consultant, Oral and Maxillofacial/Head and Neck and Reconstructive Surgeon*
- Shaukat Khanum Memorial Cancer Hospital and Research Centre, Lahore, Pakistan
- Director, Head and Neck Fellowship Program, SKMCH&RC
- Vice President, Pakistan Head and Neck Society (PHNS)

With over two decades of experience in managing complex head and neck cancers, Dr. Raza Hussain has skillfully navigated the challenges of treating cancer patients in an economically constrained environment, balancing limited resources with a high patient load. He has been involved in training postgraduate trainees and fellows, lecturing and raising awareness for oral cancer in the community, conducting hands-on live surgery courses, and publishing research in peer-reviewed journals.

Mr. Michael Gilhooly, BDS, FDSRCS, MBChB, FRCS

- *Consultant, Oral and Maxillofacial/Head and Neck and Reconstructive Surgeon*
- London Northwest University NHS Trust, London, United Kingdom

With a career spanning over three decades, Mr. Michael Gilhooly has served as a Consultant in Oral and Maxillofacial Surgery (OMFS)/Head and Neck Surgery. He is recognized as a trailblazer in modern microvascular surgery within the northwest London region, having established his own surgical unit and contributing to the training of surgeons throughout his distinguished journey.

CHAPTER 1

Buccal Mucosa

KEY POINTS

- **Aggressive Tumor Management**: Buccal mucosa cancer is aggressive, with a high rate of locoregional spread, necessitating wide local excision and selective neck dissection to control lymphatic spread and reduce recurrence risk.
- **Complex Anatomical Considerations**: The intricate buccal anatomy involves the following structures: the buccinator muscle, parotid duct, facial artery, and accompanying vein and facial nerve. It requires precise surgical planning to balance cancer control with preservation of essential functions, such as speech and mastication.
- **Reconstructive Techniques**: Reconstruction is tailored to defect size. Small defects are often closed using local tissue (buccal fat pads), while larger defects may require submental or nasolabial flaps, and extensive defects often utilize free flaps like the radial forearm for optimal restoration of function and aesthetics.
- **Post-Operative Care**: Jaw physiotherapy is critical post-surgery to prevent trismus and optimize long-term functional outcomes, especially for those cases where adjuvant radiotherapy is administered.

Buccal mucosa cancer, a subtype of oral squamous cell carcinoma (SCC), presents unique challenges due to its aggressive behavior and high rate of locoregional spread. The complex anatomy of the buccal region includes vital structures like the buccinator muscle, Stensen's duct, and facial nerve. Surgical planning necessitates assessment of both the area and depth of invasion of the cancer to ensure both adequate resection and

DOI: 10.1201/9781032714585-1

optimum reconstruction. Treatment generally involves a combination of wide local excision and neck dissection (ND) to address potential lymphatic spread.

When considering reconstruction it is always worth resorting to "the reconstructive ladder," as there are usually several options available, depending on the site, area, and depth of the defect created. Also worth considering is the availability of excess facial/cervical skin which may be turned inward to reconstruct mucosal defects. Often the final choice of flap(s) depends on the surgeon's personal experience and preference. Nevertheless, the goals of reconstruction remain the same: the restoration of function (addressing concerns of speech, mastication, and maintaining oral competence) and obtaining a satisfactory aesthetic result.

Smaller posterior buccal defects can be closed using the buccal fat pad flap; for more anterior buccal defects, the nasolabial flap has been successfully used, while with larger and/or more complex defects, submental flaps or nasolabial flaps are frequently employed due to their proximity and favorable tissue characteristics.

As the size of the defect increases, the submental island flap (with caveats regarding nodal status – see the discussion below) tends to assume primacy over the nasolabial flap. A major advantage of the submental island flap compared to the nasolabial flap is the fact that the donor defect scar is hidden under the jawline. Often, the decision of which flap to utilize depends on the amount of skin laxity at the flap site.

Regional flaps can be employed in addition to the buccal fat pad or nasolabial flap when skin cover is necessary. Either a cervical rotation flap or a forehead flap can be raised, the factors in consideration being the availability of cervical skin and cosmesis in the case of the forehead flap.

The authors have also successfully used a double paddle pectoralis major flap in those situations where skin availability or cosmesis precluded the use of the aforementioned flaps.

Microvascular flaps such as the radial forearm or anterolateral thigh flap are reserved for extensive and/or through-and-through resections, and they are frequently used as the flaps of first choice in the Western world, where surgical facilities and a reduced patient burden exist.

Given the high recurrence rates and metastatic potential in advanced cases, post-operative radiotherapy is commonly recommended. This combined approach – surgical excision with selective ND, followed by radiotherapy – serves as the standard treatment, providing both curative and palliative outcomes depending on the disease stage.

CLINICAL CASES

Case 1.1

A 55-year-old male, betel nut user and occasional smoker presented with an ulcerative growth in the right buccal mucosa for 3 months. The biopsy revealed clinically well-differentiated SCC, with an exophytic circumscribed 3 × 2 .5 cm lesion in the right buccal mucosa with associated leukoplakia.

The MRI scan showed T3N0 disease involving buccinators and abutting orbicularis oris muscle.

After the MDT discussion, primary resection and ipsilateral ND level 1–3 along with soft tissue reconstruction was performed.

Reconstruction was performed using a submental flap based on the ipsilateral submental artery to cover the internal as well as the external defect.

Final histopathology showed pT3N2b disease with a tumor size of 3.2 cm and depth of invasion of 1.3 cm. Two of 38 lymph nodes were positive at level 1.

The patient underwent post-operative radiotherapy (PORT) and has had regular follow-ups without disease recurrence (Figures 1.1–1.5).

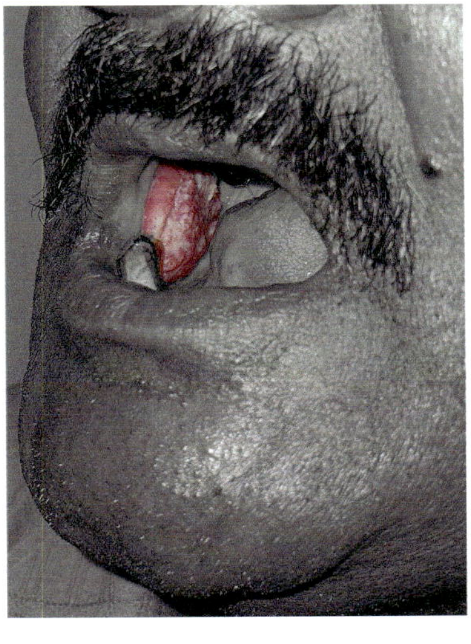

FIGURE 1.1 Right buccal mucosa SCC.

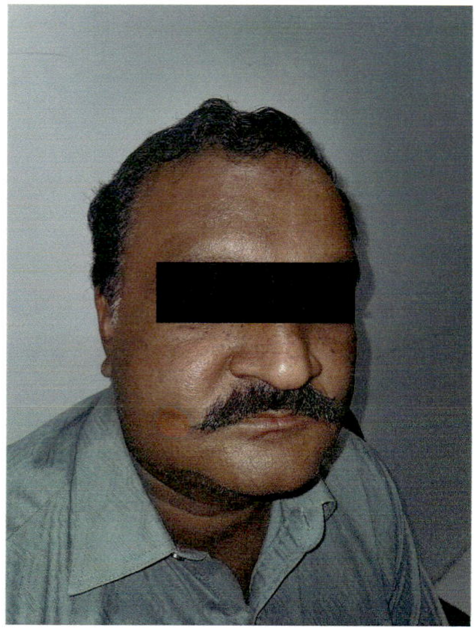

FIGURE 1.2 Subdermal extension causing skin tethering.

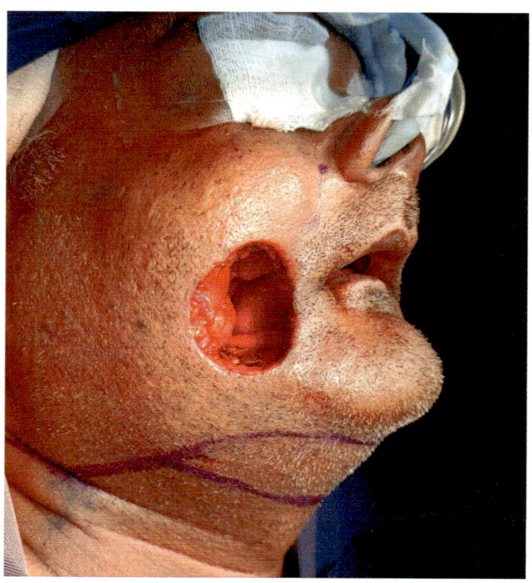

FIGURE 1.3 Through-and-through defect following resection.

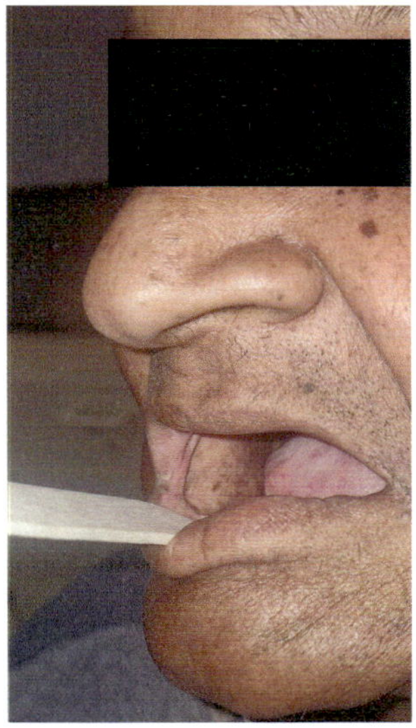

FIGURE 1.4 Post-operative submental flap.

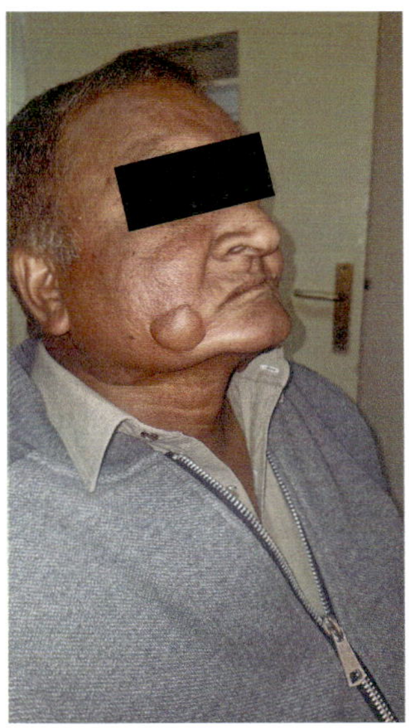

FIGURE 1.5 Post-operative external defect coverage.

Case 1.2

A 44-year-old Caucasian male presented with a small ulcer on the right buccal mucosa. No significant history of alcohol or tobacco use. Radiologically staged as T1N0M0 based on MRI of the head and neck, CT of the chest, and ultrasound of the neck.

The patient underwent wide local excision. The final staging was pT2pN1 with one positive facial lymph node. After the MDT discussion, the patient underwent post-operative radiotherapy. On follow-up, the patient developed nodal and lung metastasis and died within 18 months of diagnosis (Figures 1.6–1.8).

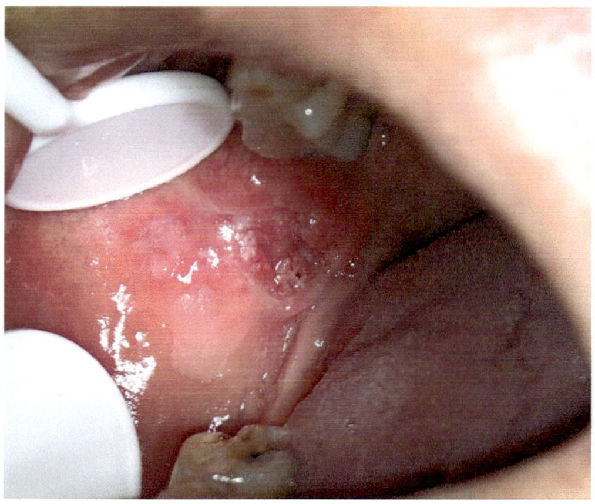

FIGURE 1.6 Small ulcer in the left buccal mucosa.

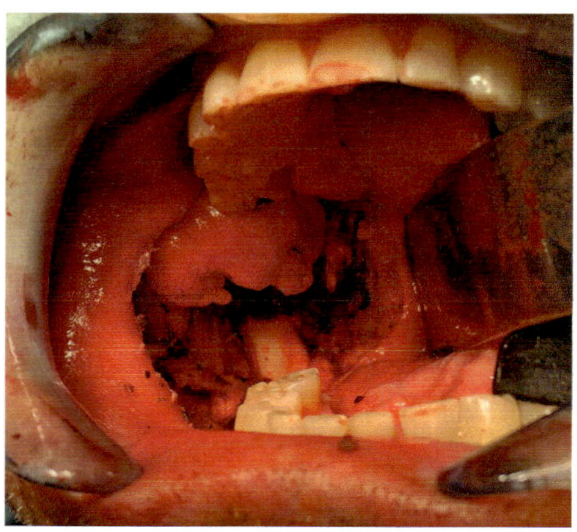

FIGURE 1.7 Wide local excision with 1 cm margin.

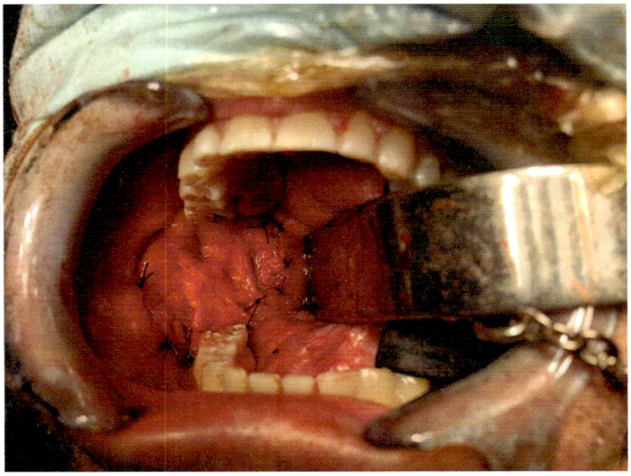

FIGURE 1.8 Buccal fat pad reconstruction.

Case 1.3

A 35-year-old male presented with right buccal mucosa SCC approaching RMT, cT2NO. We did wide local resection and two-stage nasolabial flap reconstruction (Figures 1.9 and 1.10).

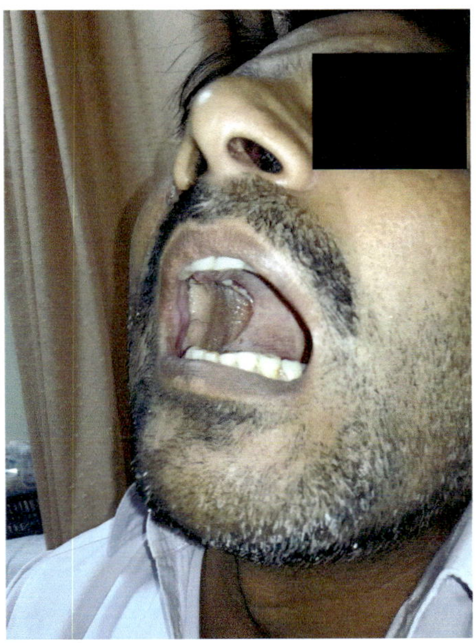

FIGURE 1.9 Nasolabial flap inset.

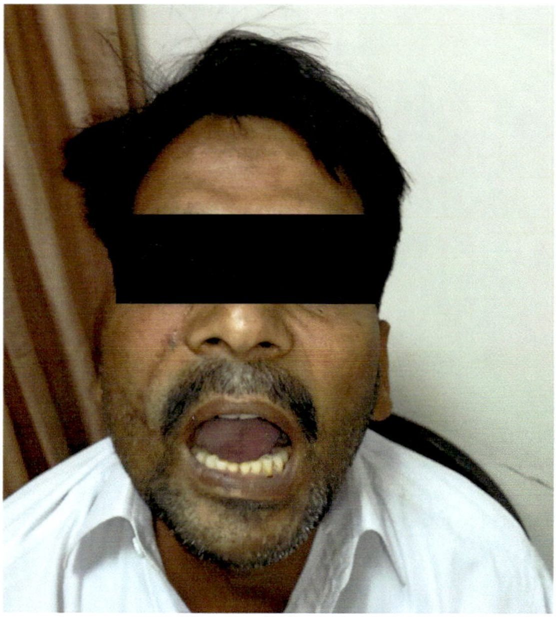

FIGURE 1.10 Good mouth opening.

Case 1.4

A 62-year-old male with T1 SCC right buccal mucosa (Figures 1.11–1.13).

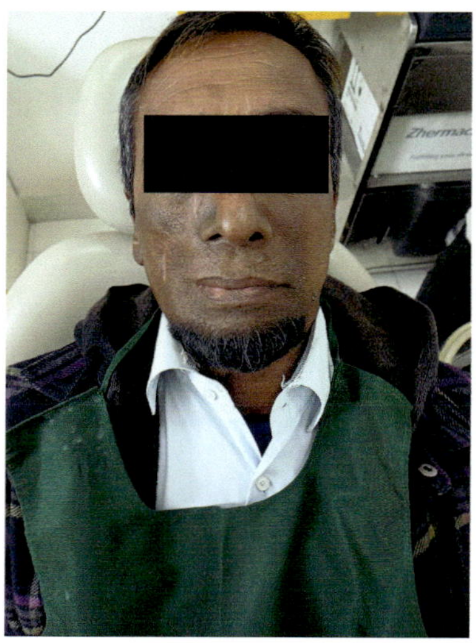

FIGURE 1.11 T1 SCC right buccal reconstructed with nasolabial flap.

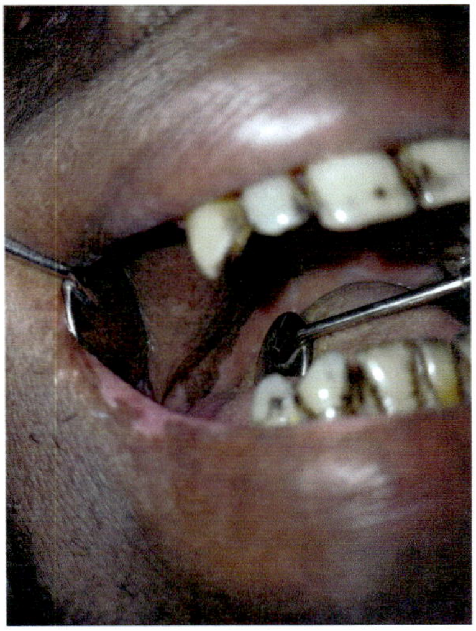

FIGURE 1.12 Intra-oral reconstruction.

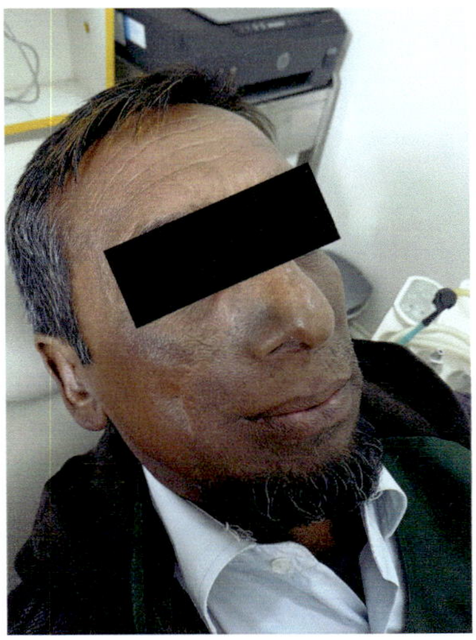

FIGURE 1.13 External scar 3 months post-operative.

Case 1.5

A 52 year old with a history of betel nut and paan use. Kept Gul (local tobacco leaf powder) in a vestibule. Reconstruction with nasolabial flap (Figures 1.14–1.18).

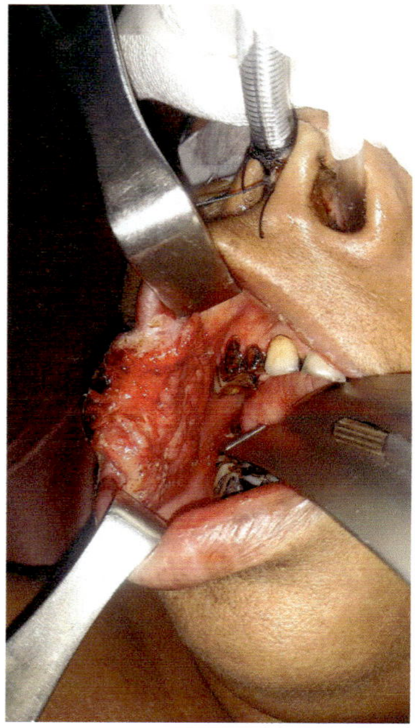

FIGURE 1.14 SCC left buccal and commissure.

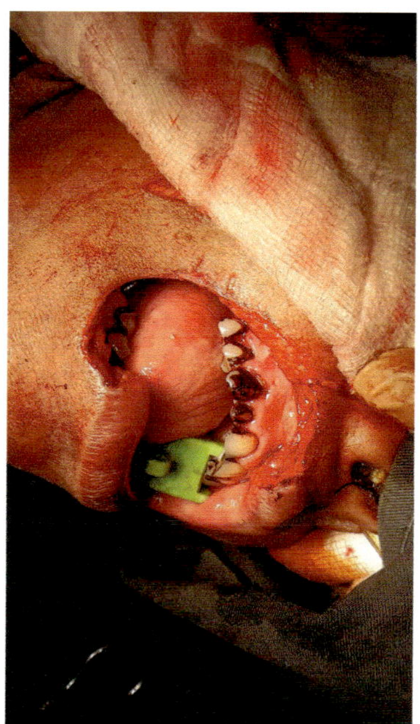

FIGURE 1.15 After resection.

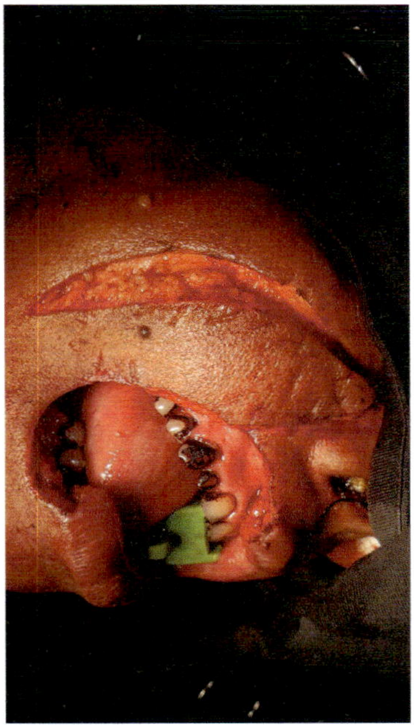

FIGURE 1.16 Inferiorly based nasolabial flap.

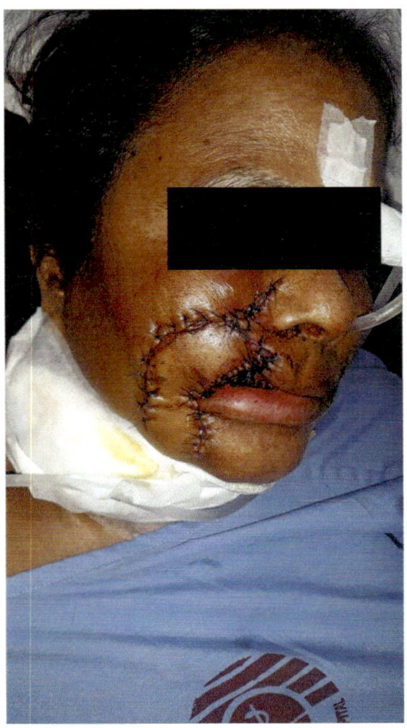

FIGURE 1.17 Immediately post-operative.

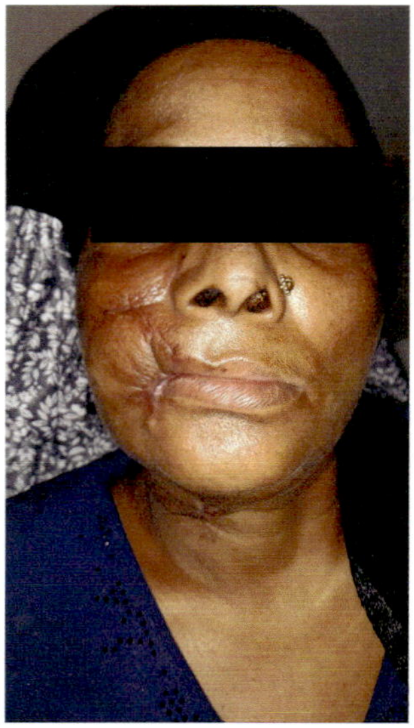

FIGURE 1.18 Several months later.

Case 1.6

A 65-year-old patient with SCC of the right buccal mucosa involving the attached gingiva (Figures 1.19–1.23).

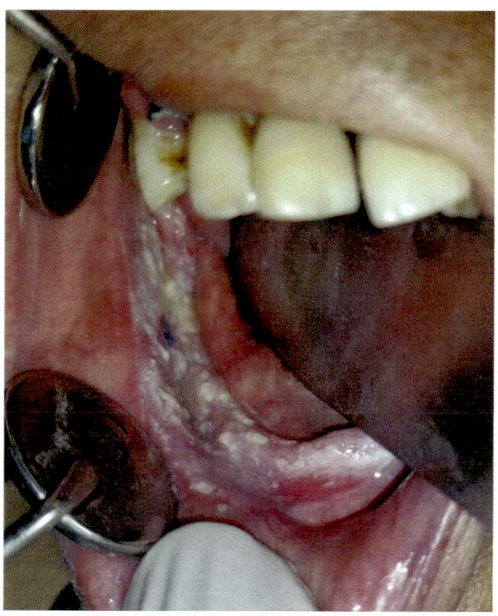

FIGURE 1.19 SCC left buccal mucosa.

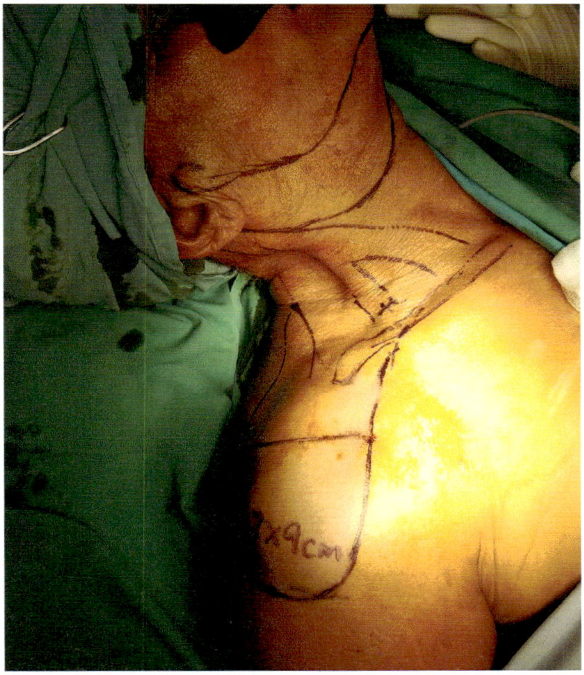

FIGURE 1.20 Through-and-through defect outlined.

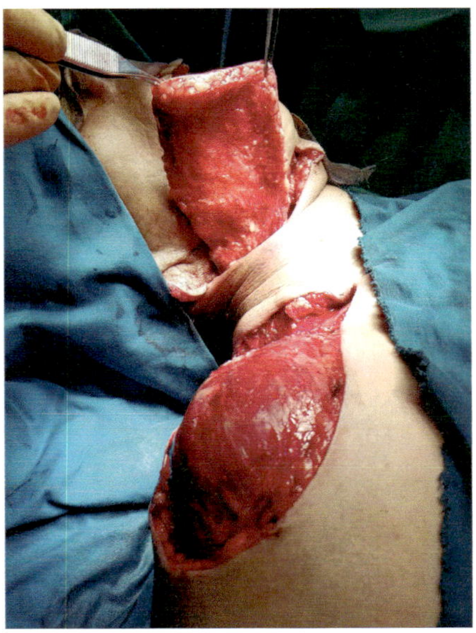

FIGURE 1.21 Defect with segmental mandibulectomy.

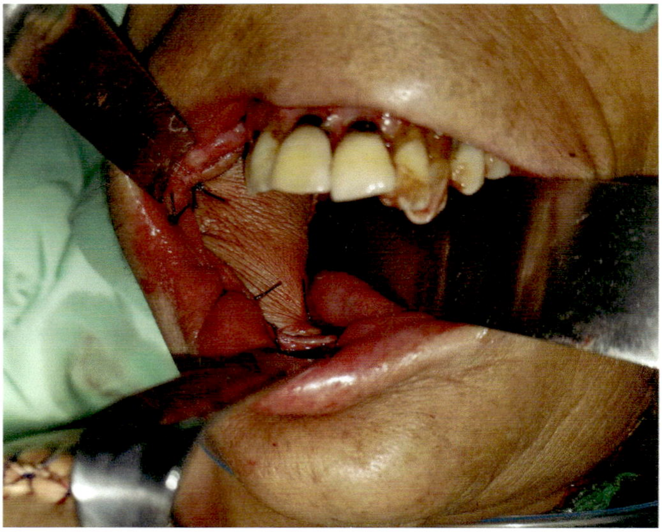

FIGURE 1.22 Immediately post-reconstruction with a pectoralis major flap.

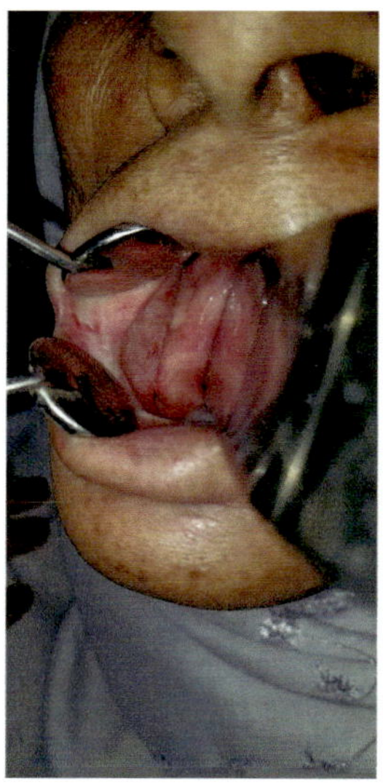

FIGURE 1.23 Three months post-operative.

Case 1.7

A 68 year old with SCC left buccal mucosa (T2N0) underwent wide local excision and reconstruction with a temporalis flap (Figures 1.24–1.28).

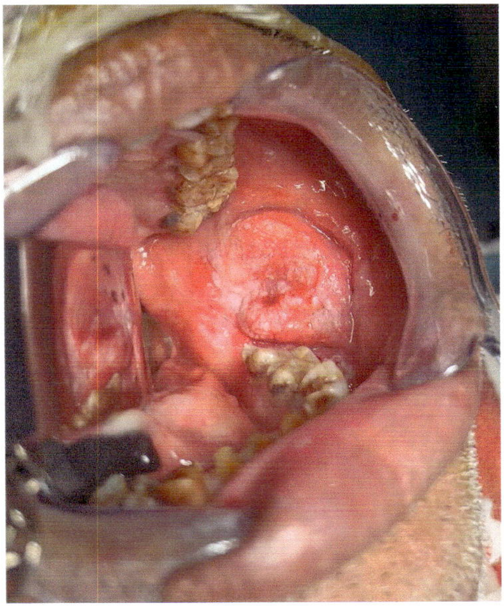

FIGURE 1.24 SCC left buccal mucosa.

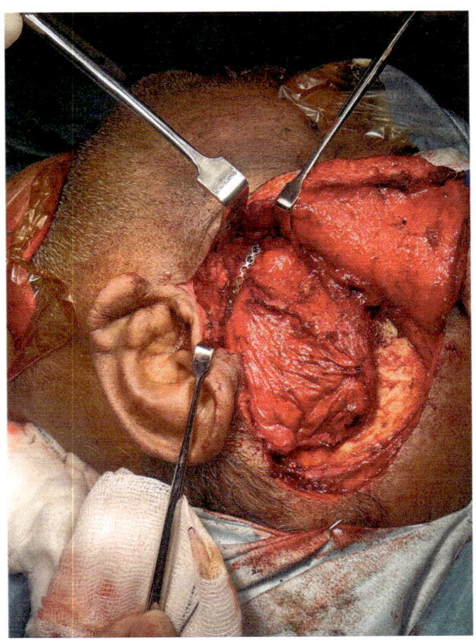

FIGURE 1.25 Temporalis flap raised and zygomatic osteotomy site pre-plated.

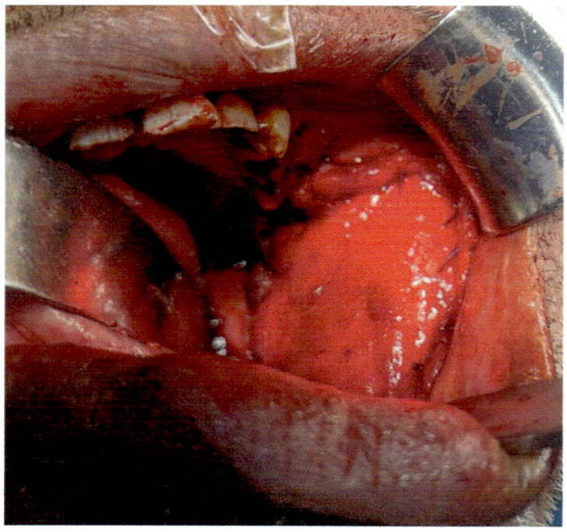

FIGURE 1.26 Temporalis flap inset.

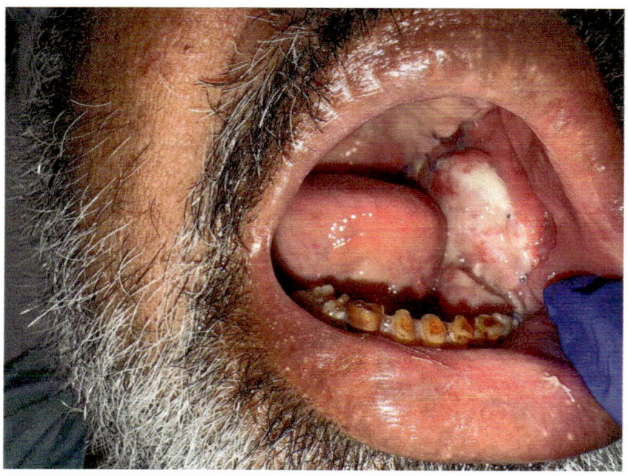

FIGURE 1.27 Three weeks post-operative.

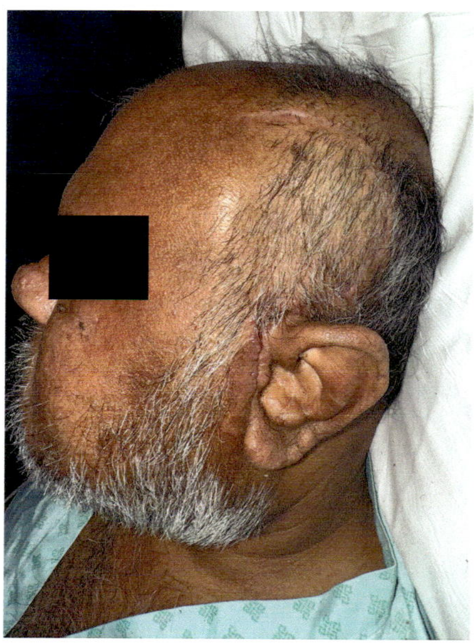

FIGURE 1.28 Temporal wound 3 weeks post-operative.

Case 1.8

A 32-year-old male treated for SCC lower alveolar mucosa. Marginal mandibulectomy and ND followed by single-staged right nasolabial flap reconstruction (Figures 1.29–1.32).

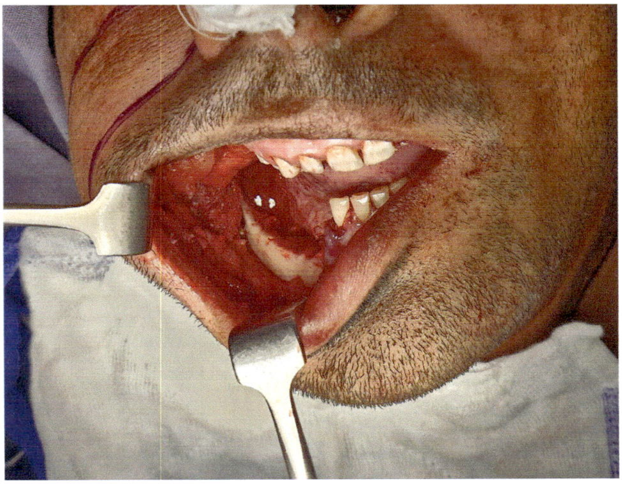

FIGURE 1.29 Wide local excision of right buccal SCC and marginal mandibulectomy.

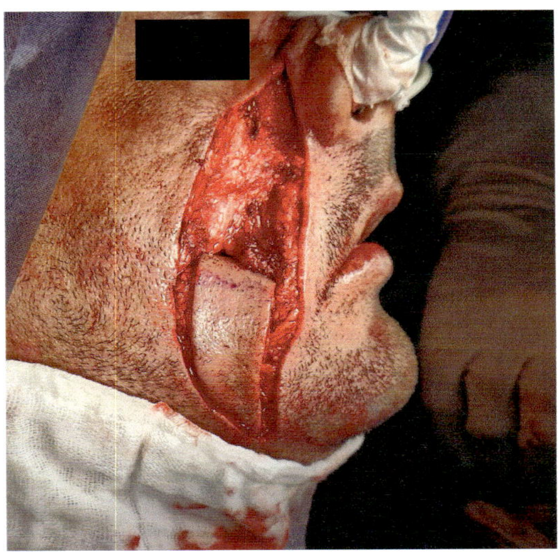

FIGURE 1.30 Nasolabial flap.

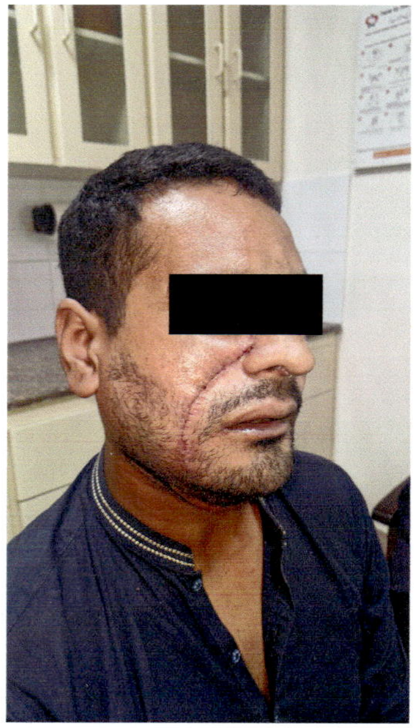

FIGURE 1.31 Post-operative nasolabial scar.

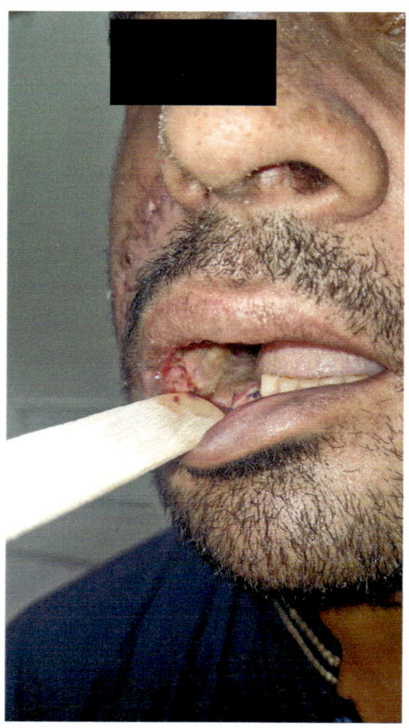

FIGURE 1.32 Intra-oral healing.

Cases 1.9 and 1.10

These cases highlight the versatility of the buccal fat pad in this region (Figures 1.33 and 1.34).

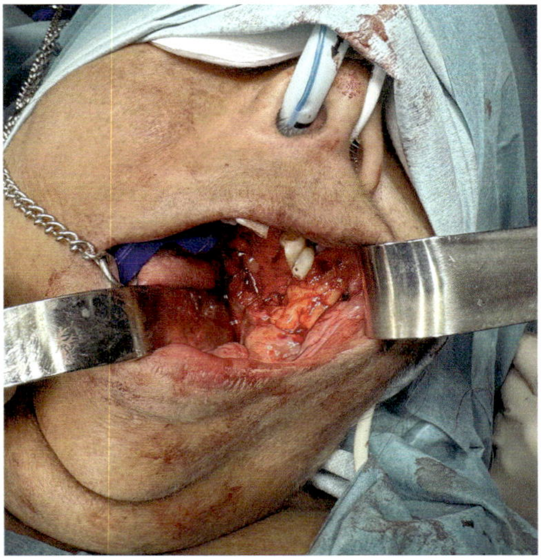

FIGURE 1.33 Left T2 SCC left buccal mucosa and retromolar area with buccal fat pad reconstruction.

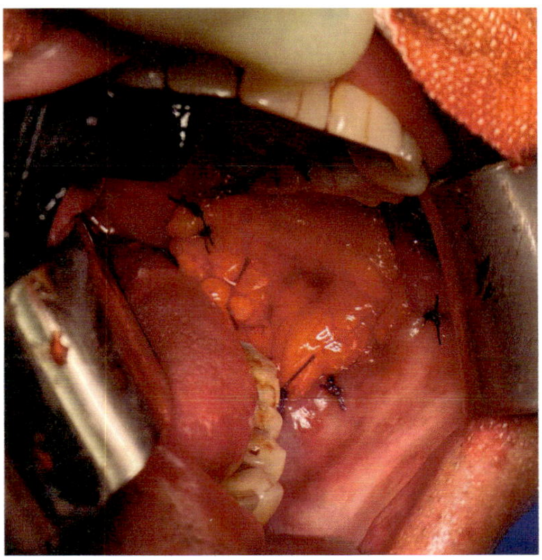

FIGURE 1.34 Small T1 posterior buccal mucosa, reconstructed with buccal fat pad.

Case 1.11

SCC right buccal mucosa with skin tethering. Underwent wide local excision through-and-through defect and reconstruction with a bi-paddled submental flap (Figures 1.35–1.38).

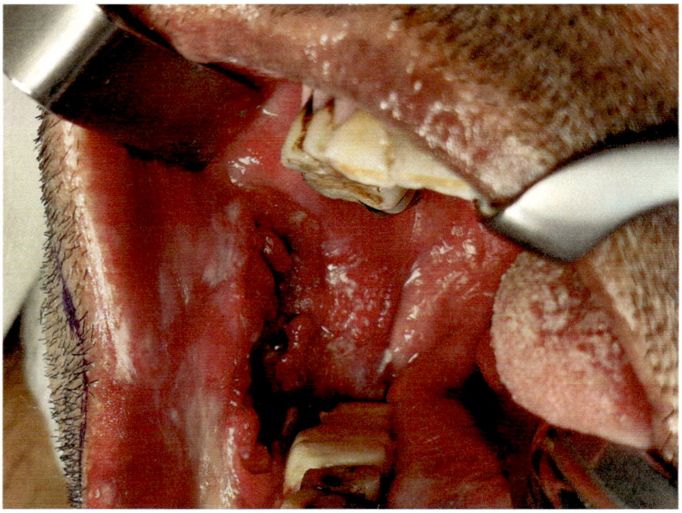

FIGURE 1.35 SCC right buccal mucosa.

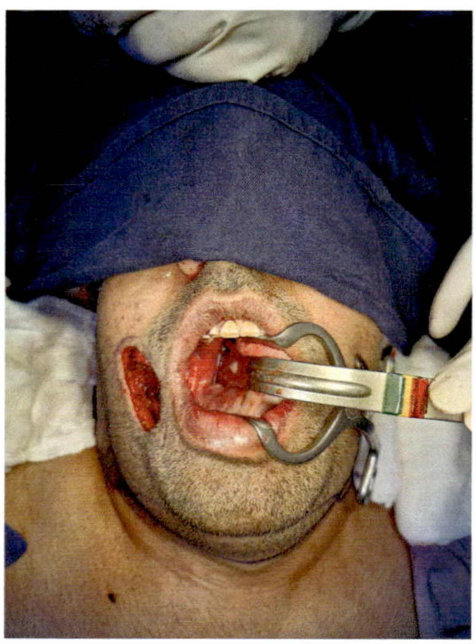

FIGURE 1.36 Excision of the tumor.

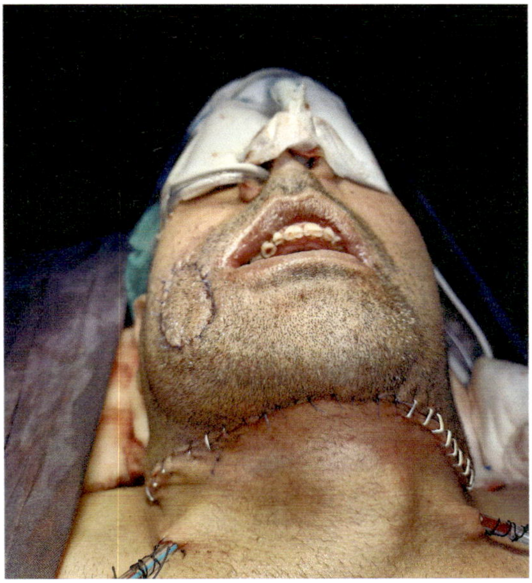

FIGURE 1.37 Reconstruction with submental flap.

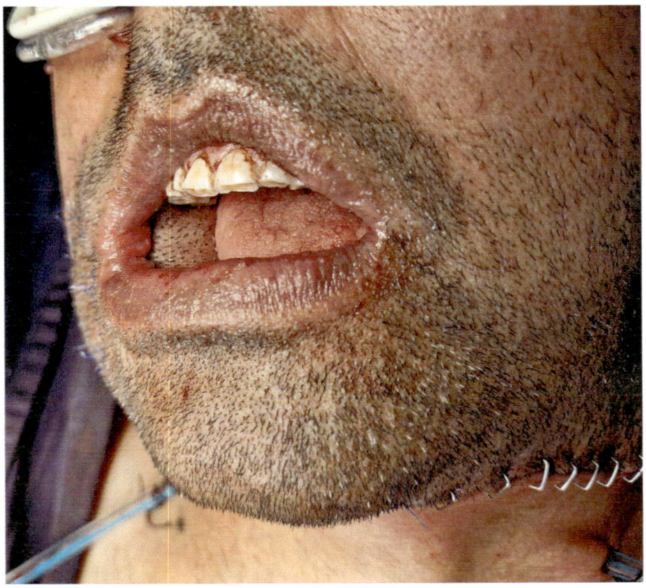

FIGURE 1.38 Bi-paddled reconstruction.

Case 1.12

SCC left buccal mucosa with commissure. Underwent reconstruction with a nasolabial flap (Figures 1.39–1.44).

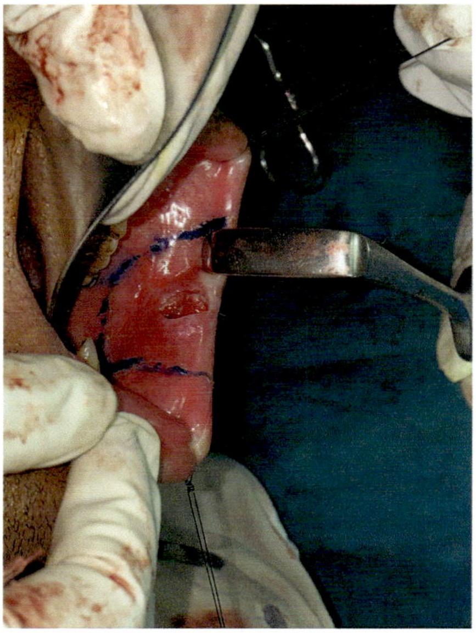

FIGURE 1.39 Buccal SCC involving commissure.

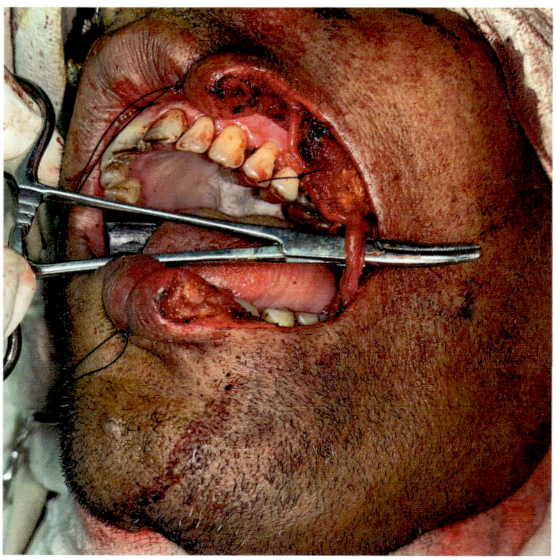

FIGURE 1.40 Wide local excision and isolation of the facial artery.

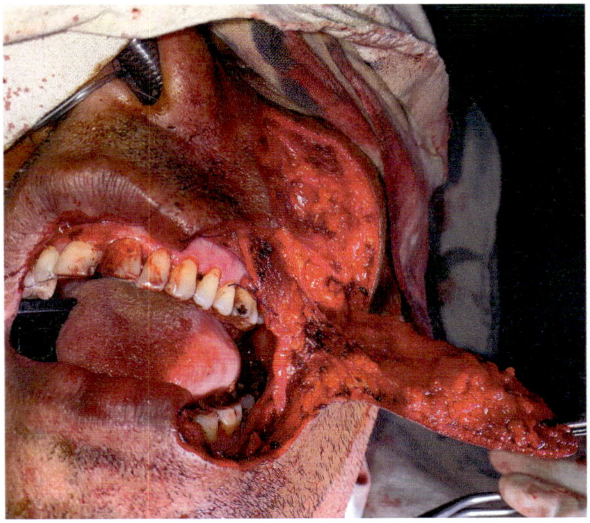

FIGURE 1.41 Nasolabial flap raised.

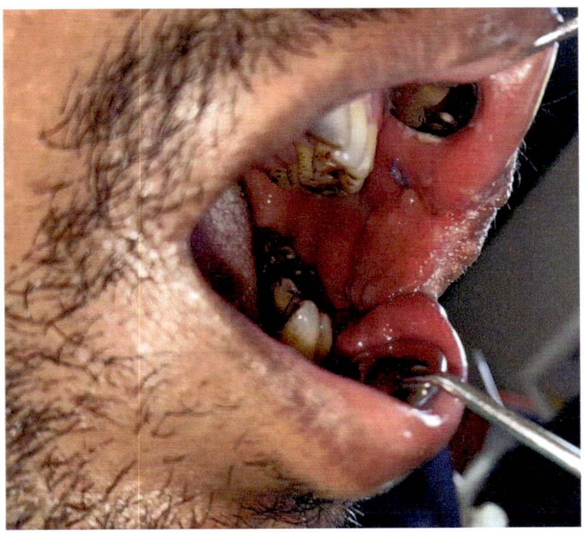

FIGURE 1.42 Inset of the flap.

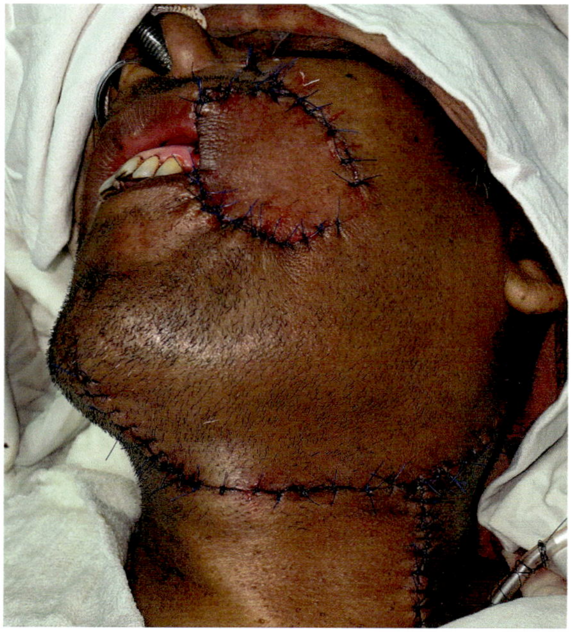

FIGURE 1.43 Defect several weeks post-operative.

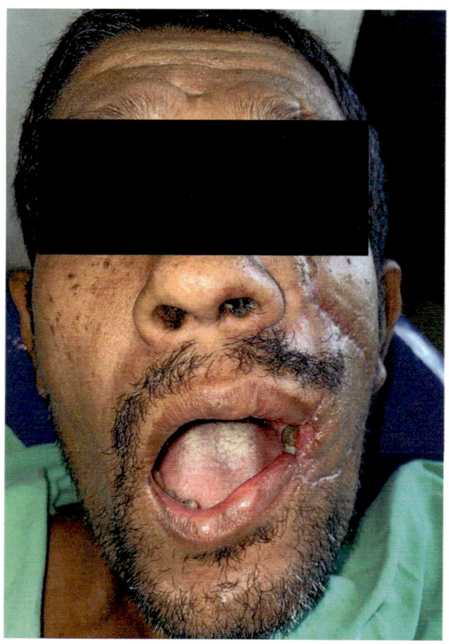

FIGURE 1.44 Good mouth opening and oral seal.

Case 1.13

SCC left buccal mucosa, reconstructed with a nasolabial flap (Figures 1.45–1.50).

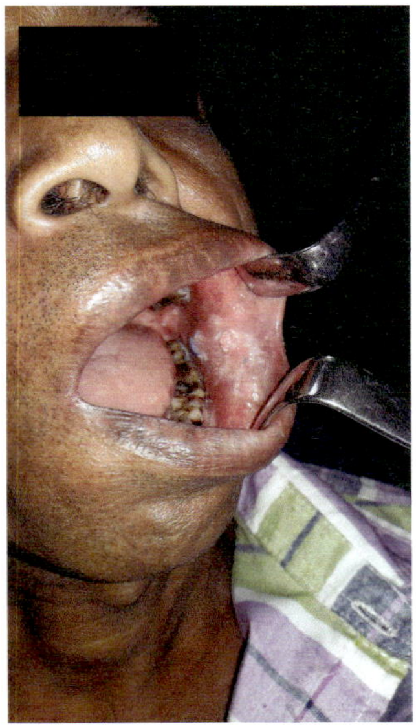

FIGURE 1.45 SCC left buccal mucosa.

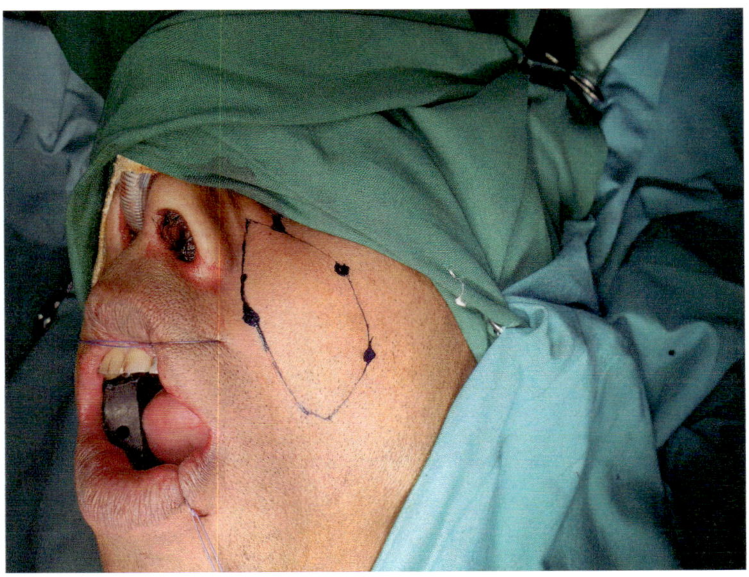

FIGURE 1.46 Nasolabial flap marking.

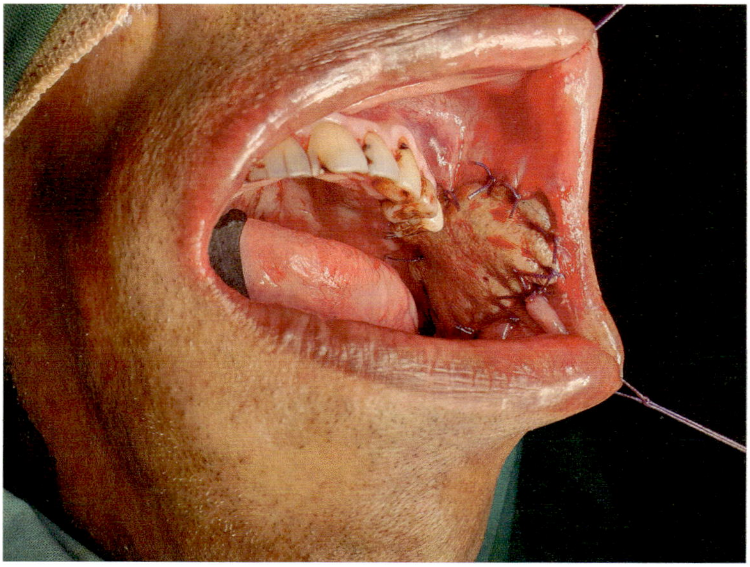

FIGURE 1.47 Flap inset.

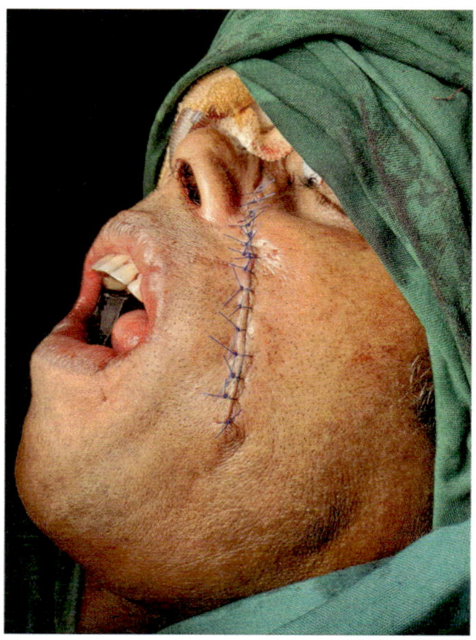

FIGURE 1.48 Donor site closure.

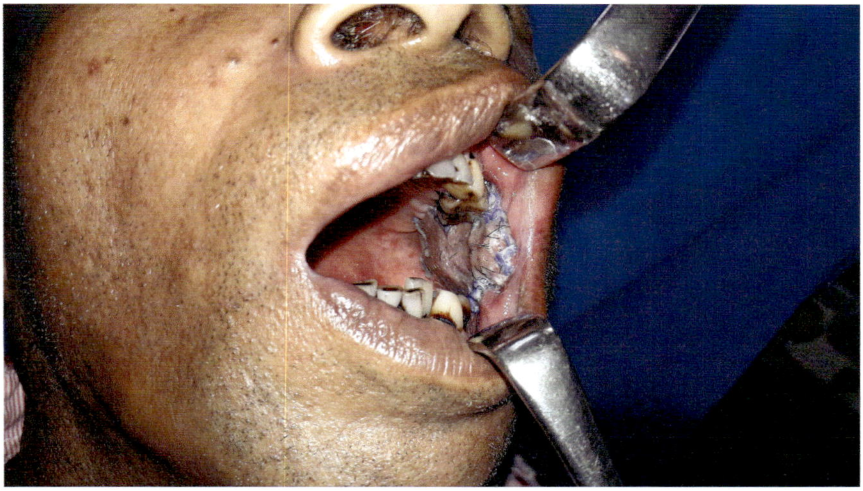

FIGURE 1.49 Several weeks post-operative. Hair growth can be seen.

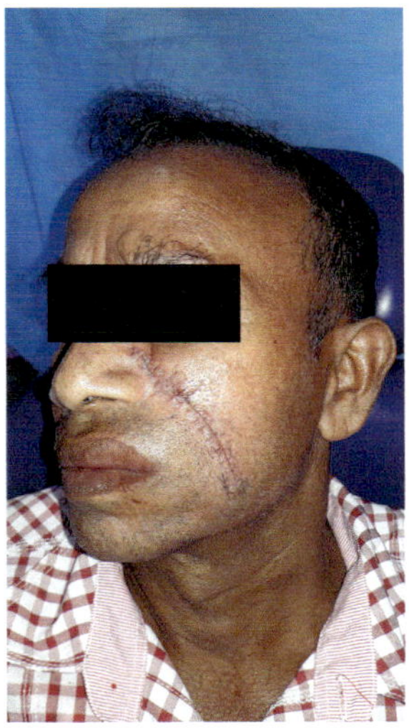

FIGURE 1.50 Post-operative donor site scar.

Case 1.14

T2 SCC of the left buccal mucosa. Underwent lip split, wide local excision, and ND. Reconstruction with platysma flap (Figures 1.51–1.56).

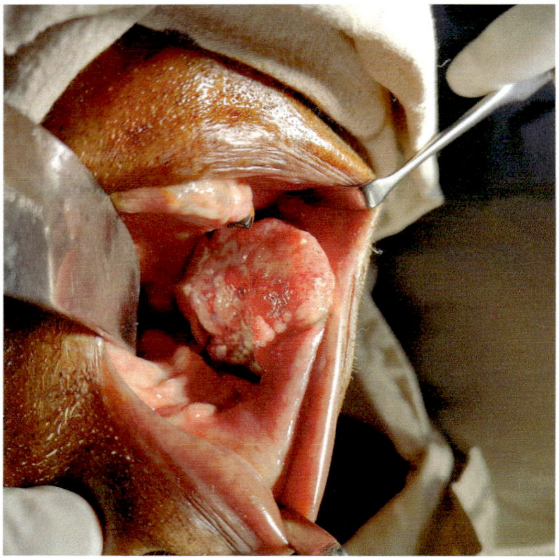

FIGURE 1.51 T2 SCC left buccal mucosa.

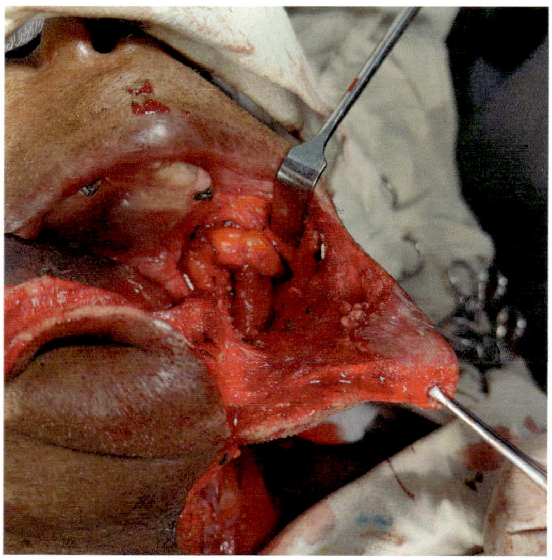

FIGURE 1.52 Lip split for access and wide local excision.

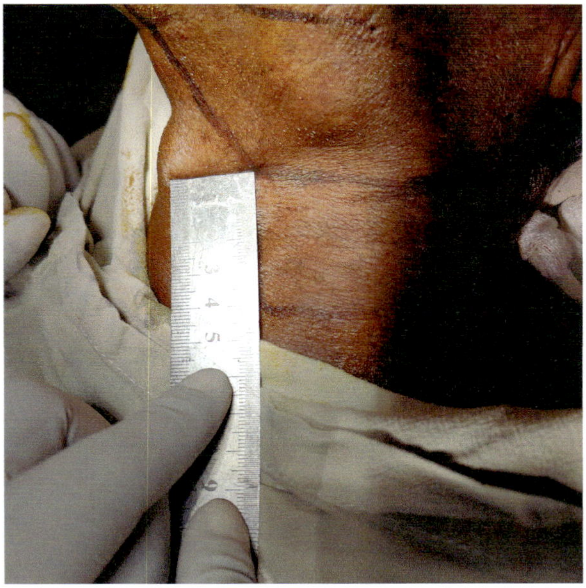

FIGURE 1.53 Platysma flap design.

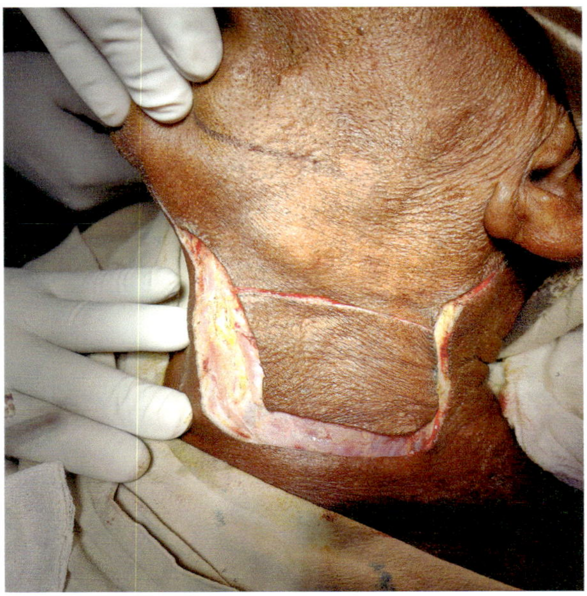

FIGURE 1.54 Platysma flap being raised.

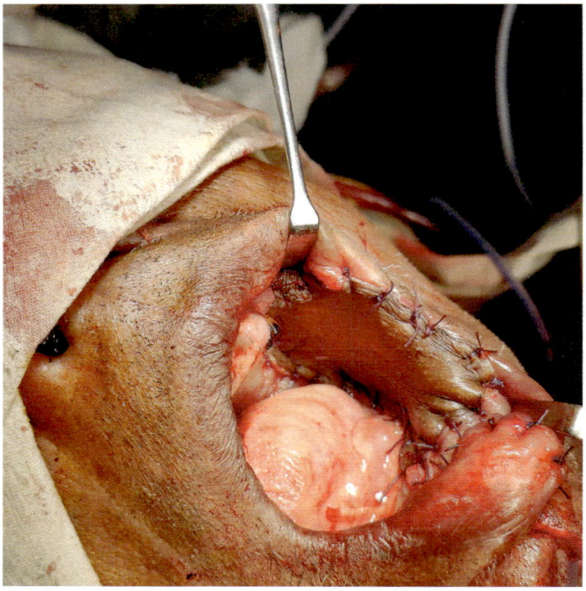

FIGURE 1.55 Flap inset.

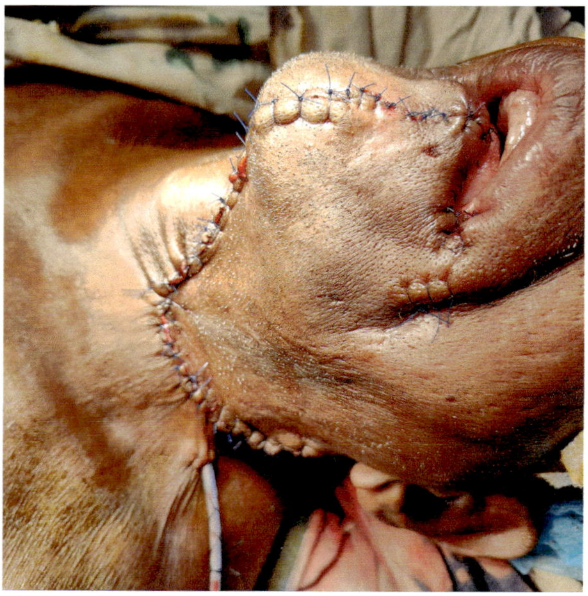

FIGURE 1.56 Donor site and neck closure.

Case 1.15

Right buccal mucosa tumor in a 58 year old with extension to the commissure. Wide local excision following reconstruction using one-stage nasolabial flap. Proximal part de-epithelialized, and primary closure done for the donor site (Figures 1.57–1.61).

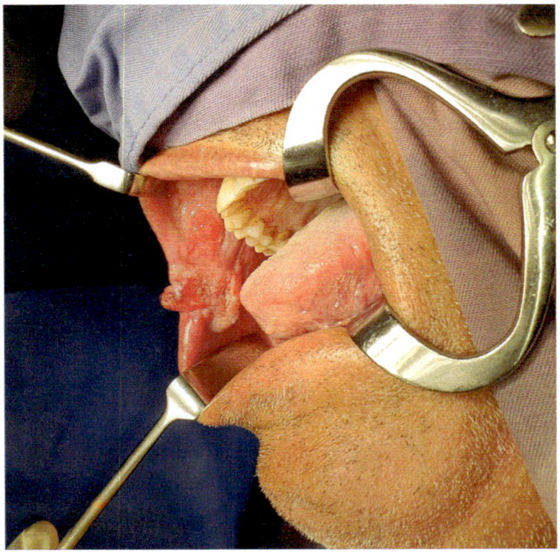

FIGURE 1.57 SCC right commissure and buccal mucosa.

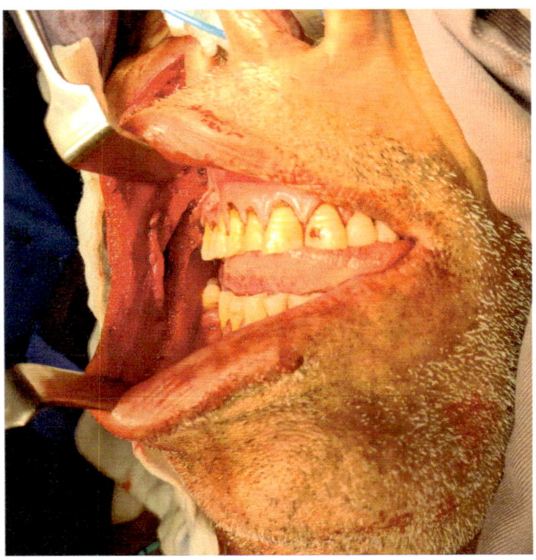

FIGURE 1.58 Wide local excision.

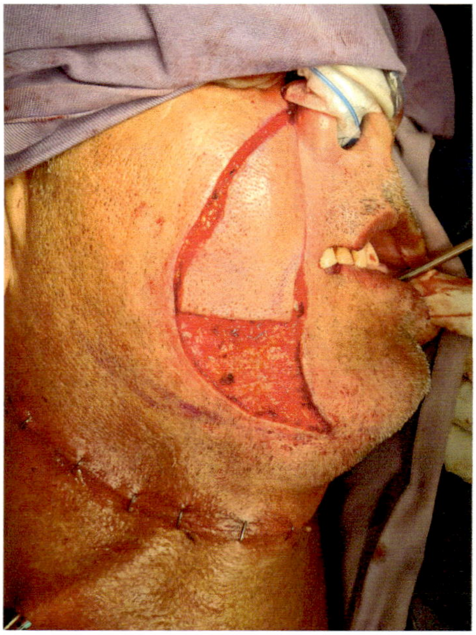

FIGURE 1.59 Nasolabial flap partially raised.

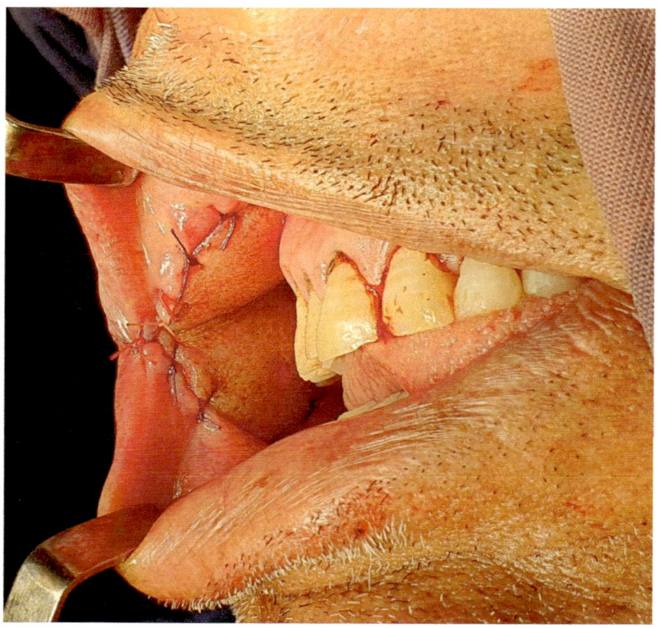

FIGURE 1.60 Flap inset.

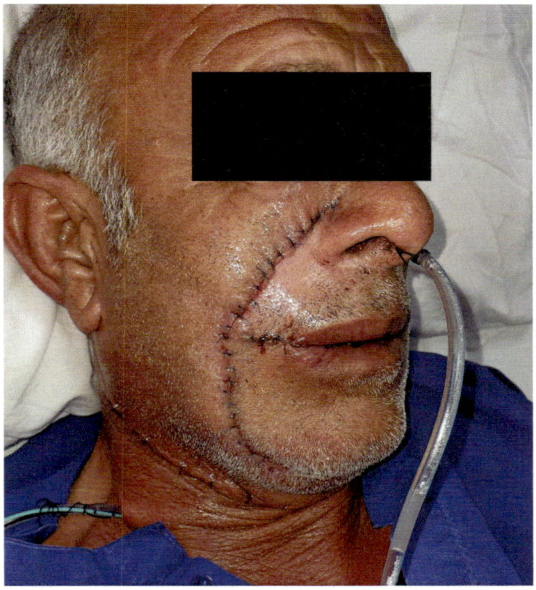

FIGURE 1.61 External wound, a few days post-operative.

DISCUSSION

In our experience managing buccal squamous cell carcinoma, particularly in populations with high incidences due to betel nut use and associated conditions such as oral submucous fibrosis (OSF), we find several common challenges and agreed-upon approaches to treatment.

Buccal squamous cell carcinoma tends to be aggressive, with a high rate of locoregional spread and poor survival outcomes. This necessitates a proactive approach with a combination of surgical resection and adjuvant radiotherapy in most cases. Surgical excision is typically wide, with selective ND (levels 1–3) based on the extent of lymph node involvement. It is necessary to include the facial lymph node in the resection.

When there is skin tethering or subdermal fat involvement, the tumor is upgraded to stage 4, necessitating full-thickness resection of the mucosa and buccinator muscle. Skin and dental extractions may also be required.

Submucous fibrosis, which frequently complicates access and assessment, adds to the difficulty of tumor resection and often exacerbates post-operative trismus. The parotid duct should be ligated during surgery to prevent complications such as sialocele or fistula, especially in cases where adjuvant radiotherapy is likely to render the parotid gland non-functional.

In patients presenting with OSF and extreme trismus (less than 1 cm mouth opening in some cases), exposure and access become critical issues. The surgeon must be cautious during tumor resection to avoid further restriction of mouth opening, which would significantly impair post-operative function and quality of life.

There is consensus that reconstruction should be tailored to the size and location of the defect. For smaller defects not involving the buccinator muscle, the buccal fat pad is often sufficient for closure, provided it offers adequate volume. When the fat pad is insufficient, white head varnish packing for up to 14 days can be used to support secondary healing. For medium to large defects, the submental flap has proven itself to be reliable and provides sufficient volume to achieve tension-free closure. However, some concerns remain about oncological safety due to the potential for transferring occult disease to the recipient site. While our extended follow-up data show relatively low recurrence rates, we remain vigilant, particularly in cases where positive level 1 lymph nodes are present.

A nasolabial flap may be used for intra-oral defects, offering good cosmetic results with minimal scarring. For larger defects that involve the commissure, retromolar trigone, or alveolar mucosa, more complex reconstructions using multiple flaps or a combination of free and pedicle flaps are often required. In older patients with ample facial skin, the nasolabial flap remains a good option, though in younger patients, we prefer the submental or supraclavicular flap for optimal results.

Long-term follow-up and jaw physio-post-operative management includes aggressive jaw physiotherapy to maintain the mouth opening in an attempt to prevent trismus from developing. Patient compliance with physiotherapy can significantly impact outcomes; unfortunately, poor compliance remains a challenge in many cases.

CHAPTER 2

Tongue

KEY POINTS

- **Complex Anatomy and Functional Importance**: The tongue's role in speech, swallowing, and taste makes its cancers particularly challenging to manage. Treatment requires preserving as much function as possible while achieving effective oncologic control.
- **Defect Evaluation**: Key factors in evaluating a defect include the size, involvement of intrinsic or extrinsic muscles, and proximity to adjacent structures such as the floor of the mouth or mylohyoid muscle. These elements guide the surgical and reconstructive approaches.
- **Primary Treatment Strategy**: Surgical resection remains the cornerstone of treatment, often accompanied by neck dissection due to the high risk of lymph node metastasis. Tumor thickness is a crucial predictor for nodal involvement, influencing surgical planning.
- **Reconstructive Options**: Reconstruction after resection is vital to restore functionality and aesthetics. Options range from healing by secondary intention for small defects to advanced flaps like the submental island flap or radial forearm flap for larger, more complex defects.
- **Controversies in Management**: Certain aspects, such as the necessity of elective neck dissection in early-stage disease and the use of adjuvant radiotherapy, remain areas of debate. These decisions are often personalized, weighing the risks and benefits for each patient.

DOI: 10.1201/9781032714585-2

The management of tongue cancers presents a unique set of challenges due to the complex anatomy of the tongue and its critical roles in speech, swallowing, and taste. Cancers in this region often require a multidisciplinary approach involving head and neck surgeons, oncologists, radiologists, and reconstructive specialists to balance oncologic control with functional preservation and quality of life.

KEY ASPECTS OF DEFECT EVALUATION

Effective management of tongue cancers starts with a detailed evaluation of the defect, as the extent and location of the tumor significantly influence treatment planning and outcomes. Several factors are considered during the evaluation phase:

- **Size of the Defect**: Larger defects may require more extensive reconstructive strategies to restore function and aesthetics.
- **Intrinsic vs. Extrinsic Muscle Involvement**: Tumors that invade the extrinsic muscles, which control the movement of the tongue, often result in more significant functional impairments than those limited to intrinsic muscles, which control shape.
- **Involvement of Adjacent Structures**: Tumors that extend into adjacent areas, such as the floor of the mouth (FOM), sublingual gland, or submandibular gland, necessitate a more complex surgical approach.
- **Tumor Extension and Oro-Cervical Communication**: In cases where the tumor extends to involve the mylohyoid muscle, communication between the oral cavity and cervical regions may occur after resection, which requires specific surgical considerations to prevent infection and ensure wound healing.
- **Mandibular Involvement**: If the tumor extends into the lower alveolus or mandible, a composite defect is created, impacting both oral and mandibular structures. Such cases demand an integrated reconstructive approach.
- **Anticipation of Post-Surgical Changes**: The volume of residual tongue tissue post-resection is assessed with an understanding that wound contraction will occur during healing, especially in patients who undergo adjuvant radiation therapy. Radiation increases the risk of scarring and contracture, making reconstruction a crucial step to maintain functionality.

TREATMENT AND RECONSTRUCTIVE STRATEGIES

The primary treatment for tongue cancer remains surgical resection, which often includes a neck dissection to address the high likelihood of lymph node metastasis. Tumor thickness has been identified as a critical predictor of nodal metastasis, influencing the surgical strategy and extent of resection required to achieve adequate oncologic margins. Research has shown that thicker tumors have a higher propensity for lymphatic spread, emphasizing the need for precise pre-operative assessment and planning.

Following tumor removal, reconstruction plays an essential role in restoring both the form and function of the tongue. Various reconstructive options are employed depending on the defect's characteristics. Techniques range from local flaps for smaller defects to complex free flap reconstruction, such as radial forearm or anterolateral thigh flaps, for extensive tissue loss. The choice of flap depends on the defect's location and size, and the need for restoring dynamic tongue movement.

In cases involving significant functional impairment, surgeons may use flaps with neuromuscular components to improve movement and sensation in the reconstructed tongue, aiding in speech and swallowing. Moreover, reconstructive efforts must consider the potential for radiation-induced fibrosis, which can exacerbate functional deficits post-treatment. As such, reconstructions are often planned with the goal of providing additional tissue to account for contraction over time.

RECONSTRUCTIVE OPTIONS FOR TONGUE CANCER

Reconstruction after tongue cancer resection is critical for restoring function and aesthetics. Options vary based on the defect's size, depth, and involvement of surrounding structures, as well as on the individual needs of the patient. Here are the primary reconstructive approaches:

1. **Healing by Secondary Intention**
    - Small superficial defects may be left to heal naturally by secondary intention. This treatment is typically suitable for minor resections where no vital structures are affected. While simple, this method is limited to cases where functional loss is minimal. In selected cases with superficial tumors, even with wider resections, tongue wounds can be left to heal secondarily. This would delay the healing time and potential risk of wound contracture.

The anterior ventral surface of the mobile tongue has the potential to tether to the fixed gingiva, resulting in limited mobility.

2. **Skin Grafts and Synthetic Allografts**

    - **Split-Thickness Skin Grafts (STSGs)**: For larger superficial defects, split-thickness skin grafts can provide adequate coverage, particularly when aesthetic concerns are minimal. STSGs help with epithelialization but do not restore significant structural volume, limiting their utility in areas requiring bulk. The donor site must stay immobile for good uptake. The tongue is a mobile structure with strong underlying functional musculature. The grafts are usually secured by a bismuth iodoform paraffin paste (BIPP) or white head varnish dressing.

    - **Synthetic Allografts**: In cases where autologous tissue is limited, synthetic allografts can provide temporary coverage. However, these grafts generally lack durability and may not support the functional demands of the tongue.

3. **Primary Closure**

    - Small, localized defects with minimal tissue loss can sometimes be closed directly through primary closure techniques. This option is generally limited to small resections and cases where adequate mobility and tissue elasticity allow for tension-free closure, helping to reduce scarring and preserve functionality. While planning tongue reconstruction, one must not forget the primary goal, which is to achieve intelligible speech and objective swallowing. Reconstruction mainly aims to restore tongue volume and bulk.

4. **Local Flaps**

    - Local flap techniques are often employed for moderate-sized defects that cannot be managed by primary closure. Options include buccal mucosal or facial artery-based flaps, which provide reliable vascularity and are effective for intra-oral reconstructions. Local flaps offer a balance between structural restoration and functional preservation, though they may not provide sufficient volume for larger defects. The last decade has witnessed the resurgence of local tissue flaps with an inherent benefit of cost effectiveness, decreased operating time, and shorter hospital stay.

5. **Submental Island Flap**

- The submental island flap is increasingly popular in reconstructive surgery for moderate to large tongue defects. It provides well-vascularized tissue, which can support both functional and aesthetic outcomes. This flap is particularly useful in cases where microvascular free flaps are not an option due to patient factors or resource limitations. The submental flap has shown promising outcomes for restoring speech and swallowing functions due to its pliability and adaptability. The oncologic safety has remained questionable, as there is a theoretical risk of harboring the metastatic disease from level IA and IB to the primary site, but no convincing evidence suggests increased locoregional recurrence with the use of the submental flap. It is better to avoid the use of this flap in clinically metastatic level I disease with extra-nodal spread. Even in the absence of metastatic disease, a meticulous dissection around the pedicle is mandatory to assure that no fibrofatty tissue is left behind to minimize the risk of disease transfer with the flap.

6. **Nasolabial Flap**

- The nasolabial flap is based on the facial artery and can be used as an axial, random, or island flap. The availability of abundant skin in the nasolabial area in elderly patients makes it an ideal and quick choice for oral cavity reconstruction with a good, reliable blood supply. The edentulous status of the patient makes it more suitable to be used for the FOM and lateral tongue defects. The distal end of the flap is rotated into the oral cavity to cover the lateral tongue defect and later divided after 2 weeks to close the external defect and suture the proximal part of the skin paddle with the tongue. As soon as the flap division is performed, the tongue mobility improves.

7. **Facial Artery Myomucosal Flap (FAMM)**

- FAMM has been used extensively to close the cleft palate and FOM defects. The flap comprises the mucosa, submucosa, and buccinator muscle and is based on the facial artery and submucosal venous plexus. It can be superiorly or inferiorly based with a maximum dimension of 3-4 cm. The limitation of the dimension is because of the proximity of the Stensen's duct and the inability to close the donor site primarily. The flap is transferred over the alveolus to cover the lateral tongue/FOM defects but needs division after 2 weeks. Another drawback is the potential risk of trismus if harvested beyond the above-mentioned dimensions. The FAMM flap is not a good choice to utilize in a dentate patient. It is important to have a good volume of buccal pad fat, which can be used to cover the donor site. Otherwise, a dressing can be applied to cover the raw buccal defect for 2 weeks.

8. **Palatal Island Flap**

- The palatal island flap is an optimal option to cover the posterolateral dorsum of the tongue superficial defects with reasonable outcomes. The palatal flap is a mucoperiosteal flap supplied by a greater palatine artery emerging through the greater palatine foramen that enters the palatal soft tissue. It is a thin and pliable flap with a limited arc of rotation. The extent of rotation can be increased by removing the thin posterior bony column. The donor site is either left to heal secondarily over a period of 2 to 3 weeks or covered by dressing (white head varnish/BIPP) with special instructions to stay on a fluid diet and maintain good oral hygiene for 5 to 7 days. In head and neck cancer patients who have been previously irradiated, the healing of the palatal island flap donor site can be jeopardized with an increased risk of osteoradionecrosis. When using this flap for posterior tongue reconstruction, the pedicle needs to be divided in 2 weeks to release the restriction in movement during speech and swallowing.

CLINICAL CASES

Case 2.1

A 39-year-old female with no risk factors developed a right lateral tongue 4 × 2.5 cm ulcerative lesion with a clinically palpable endophytic component crossing the midline. Primary resection has resulted in almost 40% loss of tongue volume. The submental flap was harvested and rotated through the FOM to cover the tongue defect. An acceptable bulk and adequate submental skin have permitted the restoration of the form, and the function which obviates the need for free flap reconstruction (Figures 2.1–2.6).

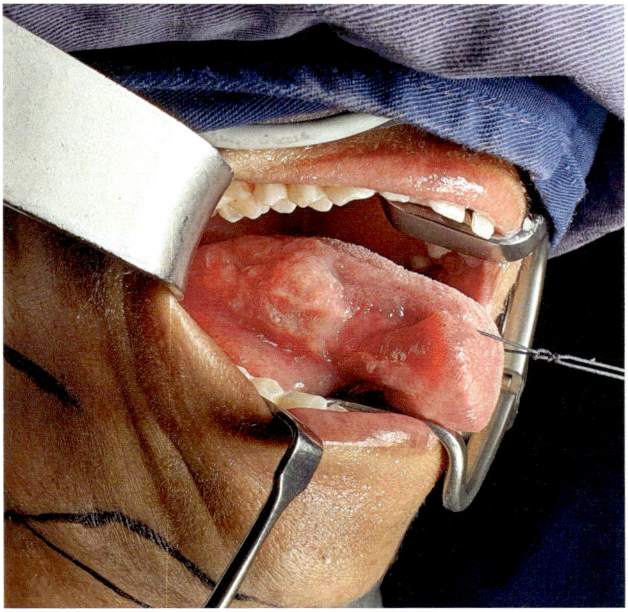

FIGURE 2.1 A right lateral tongue 4 × 2.5 cm ulcerative lesion.

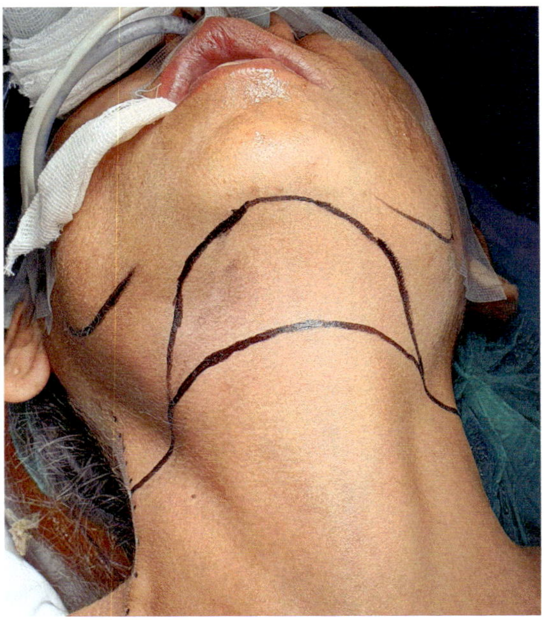

FIGURE 2.2 A submental flap marked using a "pinch" test.

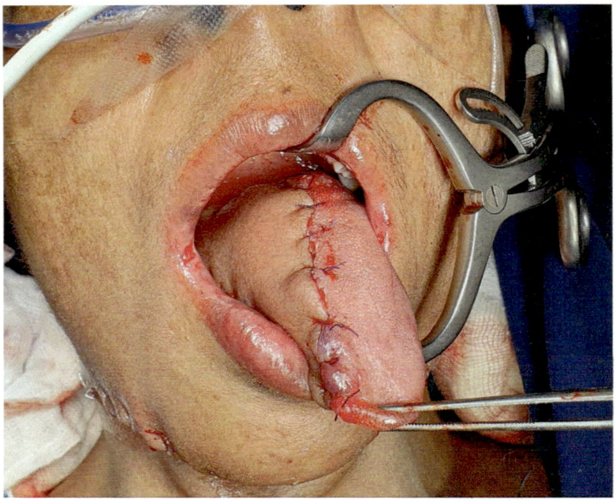

FIGURE 2.3 A flap inset into the defect, restoring a volume of resected tongue.

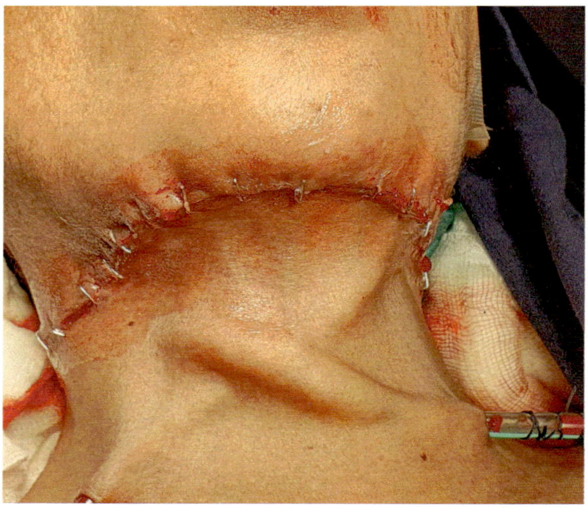

FIGURE 2.4 Primary closure of the neck wound.

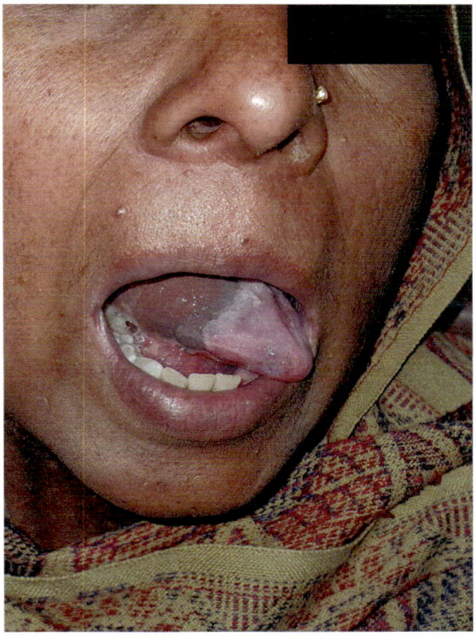

FIGURE 2.5 The tongue after radiotherapy.

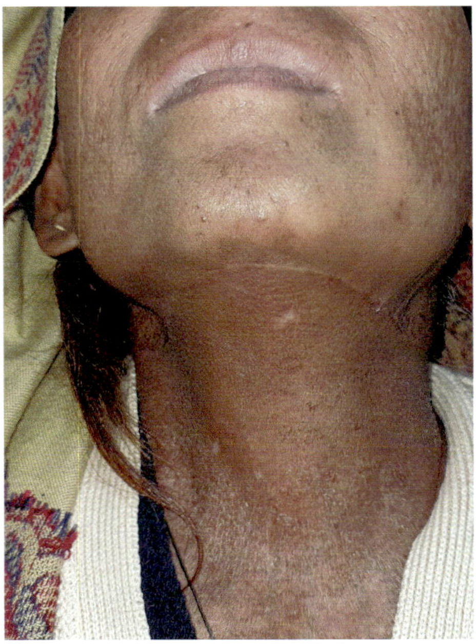

FIGURE 2.6 A submental scar 6 months after adjuvant treatment.

Case 2.2

A 48 year old with a T2 SCC left lateral tongue underwent a partial glossectomy, neck dissection, and reconstruction with a submental flap (Figures 2.7–2.9).

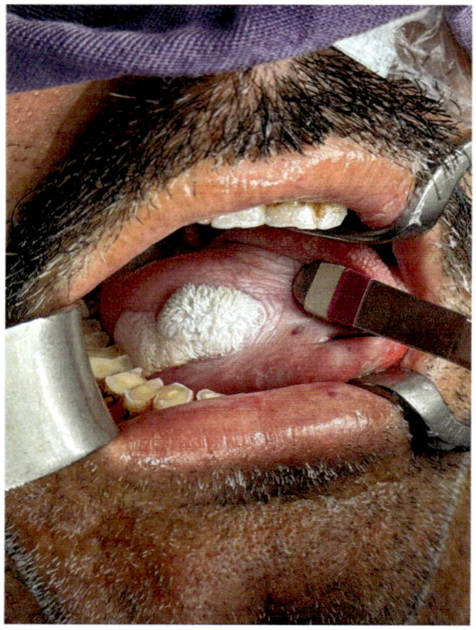

FIGURE 2.7 Right lateral whitish tongue exophytic mass.

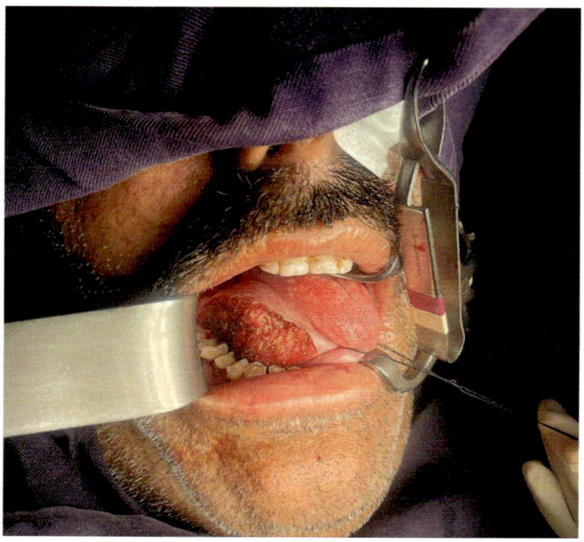

FIGURE 2.8 Excision.

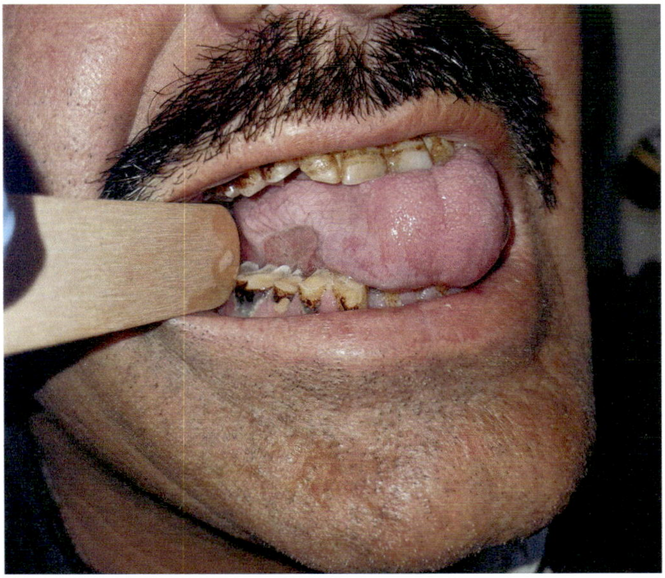

FIGURE 2.9 Well-healed 2 weeks post-operatively.

Case 2.3

A 53-year-old female was diagnosed with well-differentiated SCC of the left lateral tongue. The resection involved some parts of the intrinsic muscle but created a superficial defect that was closed primarily without it (Figures 2.10–2.12).

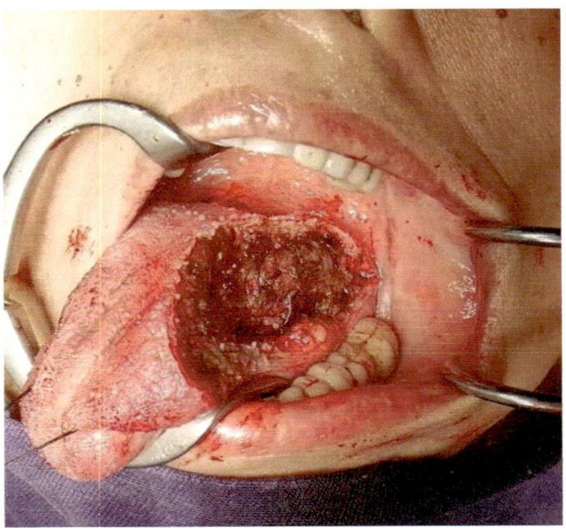

FIGURE 2.10 Left lateral defect post-resection.

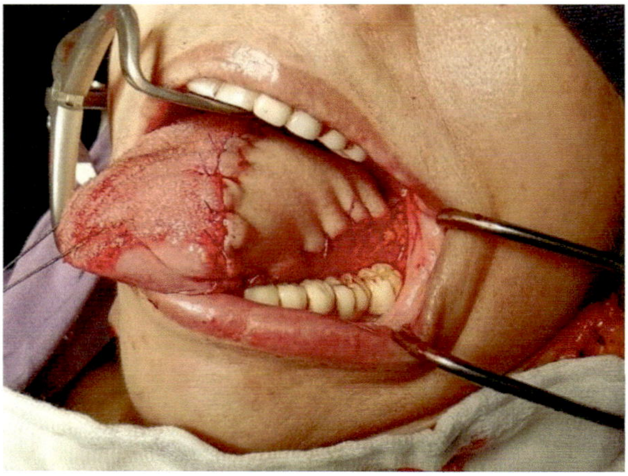

FIGURE 2.11 Reconstruction with left submental flap.

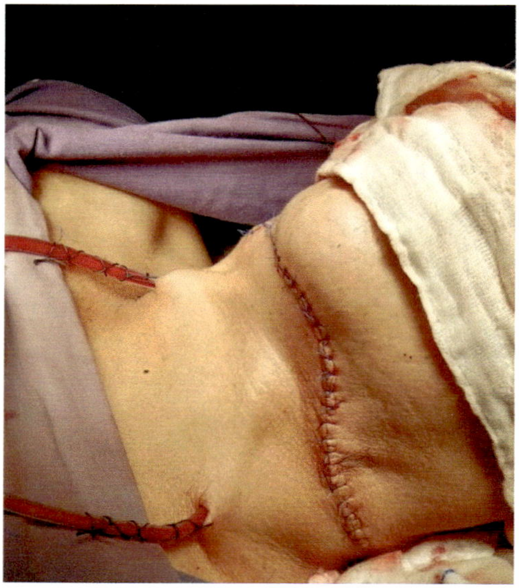

FIGURE 2.12 Neck wound.

Case 2.4

A 57-year-old male was diagnosed with SCC in the right tongue. He did not get medical clearance for long-standing surgery. The patient had poor oral hygiene and hopeless posterior dentition, which created provision for the use of a nasolabial flap. The flap was designed with an intent to have primary closure at the harvest site. After raising the flap, a tunnel was made over the risorius muscle, and the flap was rotated into the oral cavity. After 2 weeks, the flap was divided, and the external skin components as well as internal mucosal edges sutured to the adjacent skin and mucosa simultaneously (Figures 2.13–2.15).

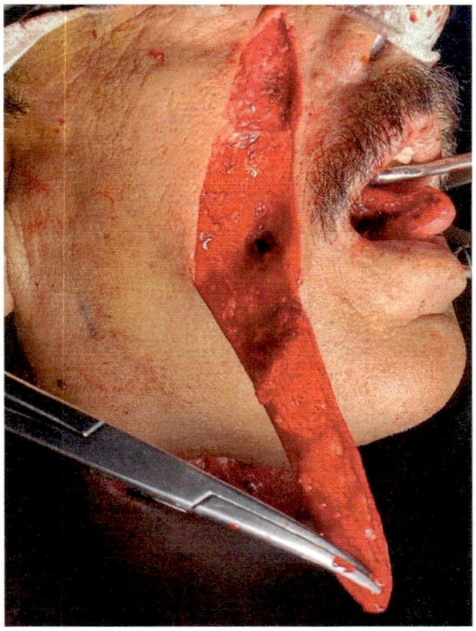

FIGURE 2.13 Right nasolabial flap raised with standard approach.

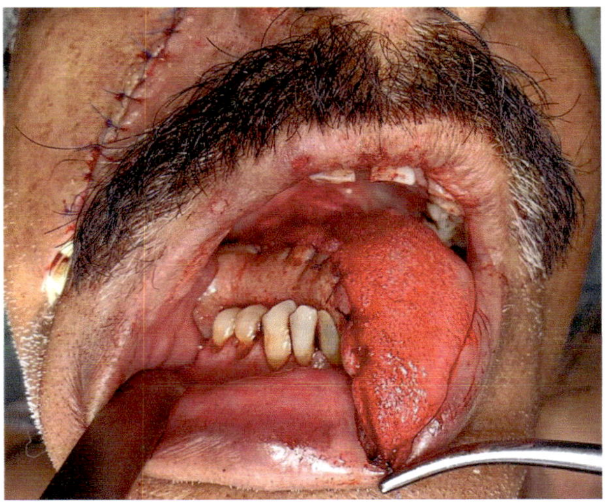

FIGURE 2.14 A tunnel created above the risorius muscle and flap rotated to cover the lateral tongue defect.

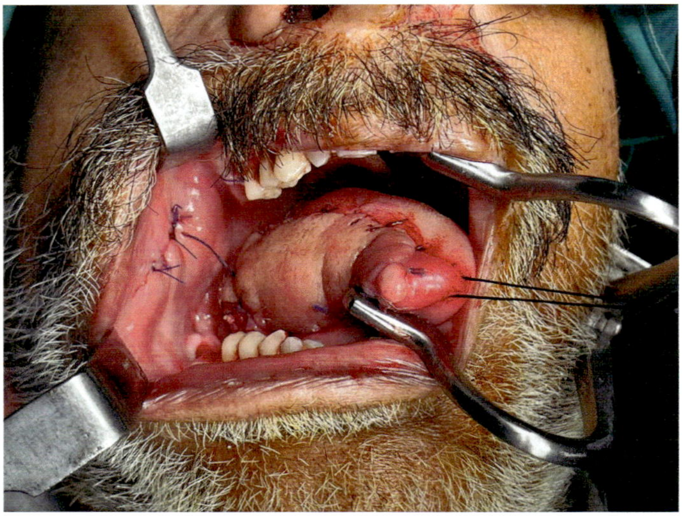

FIGURE 2.15 Division of the flap after 2 weeks. The buccal mucosa tunnel can be primarily closed.

Case 2.5

A 47 year old with large T4 SCC of the tongue underwent a subtotal glossectomy using a pull-down approach to bring the tongue into the neck, and reconstruction was done with a pec major flap (Figures 2.16 and 2.17).

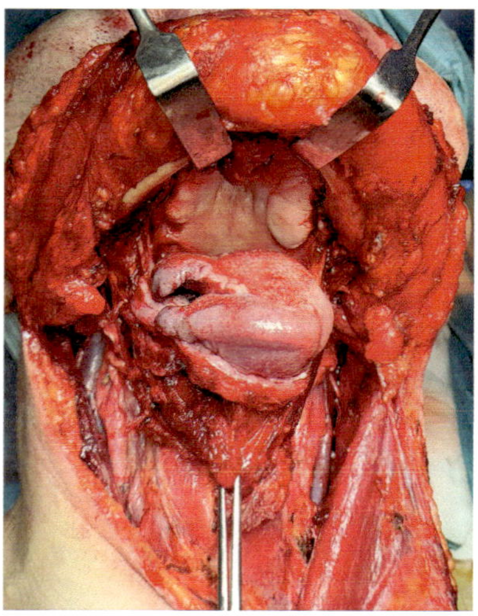

FIGURE 2.16 A large SCC T4 of the tongue crossing the midline. A cervical pull-through to expose the base of tongue.

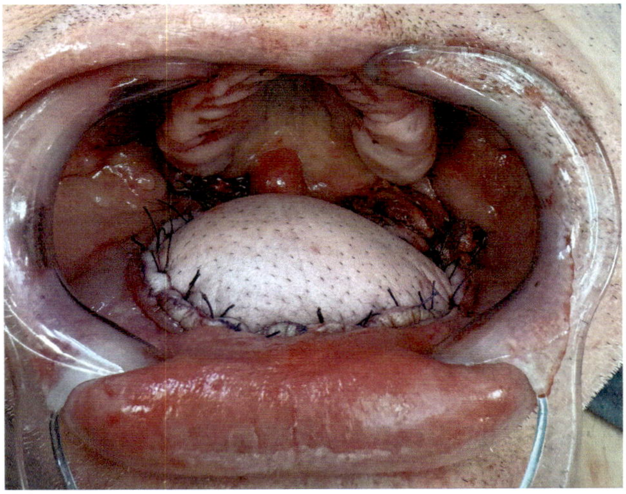

FIGURE 2.17 A pectoralis flap used to reconstruct.

Case 2.6

The patient presented with a lesion on left lateral tongue (T2N1). Following resection, the defect was reconstructed with a FAMM. The FAMM was raised fully on the pedicle and then introduced into the oral cavity on the medial aspect of the mandible. This allows it to be used in dentate patients (Figures 2.18–2.21).

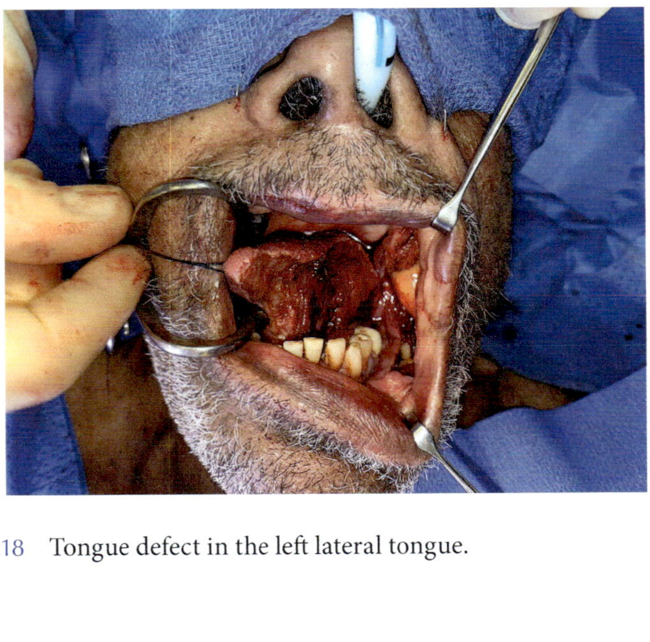

FIGURE 2.18 Tongue defect in the left lateral tongue.

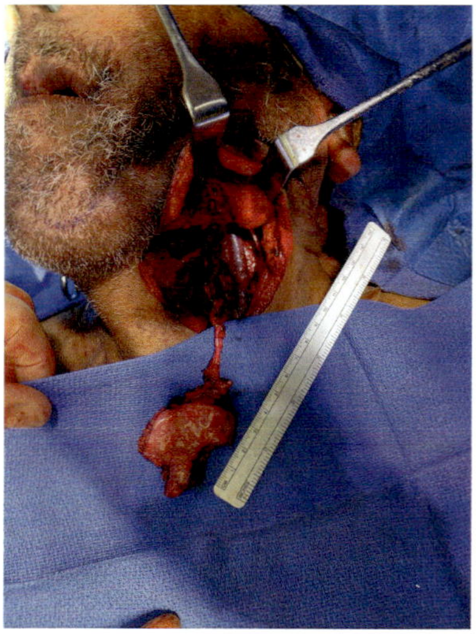

FIGURE 2.19 A FAMM flap that was raised based on the facial artery pedicle.

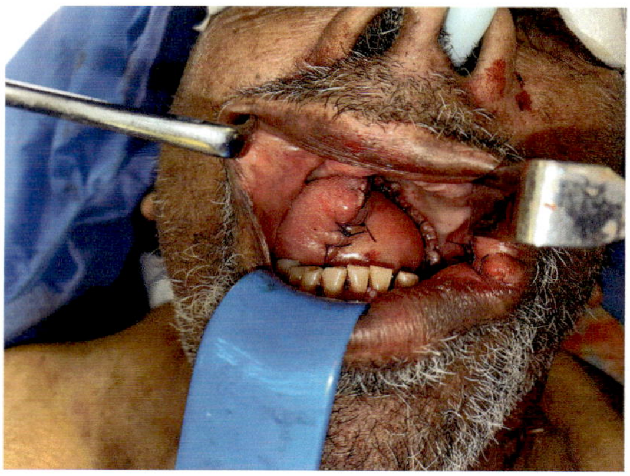

FIGURE 2.20 Flap inset.

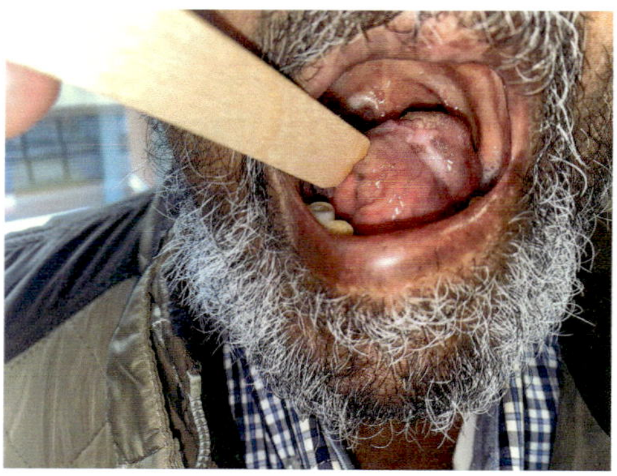

FIGURE 2.21 Flap post-operative 6 weeks later.

Case 2.7

A 70-year-old female with a T2 SCC right lateral tongue cancer underwent a partial glossectomy, right neck dissection, and reconstruction with platysma flap (Figures 2.22–2.26).

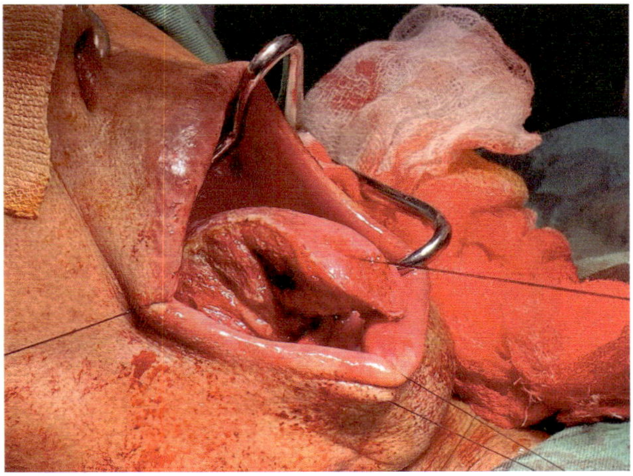

FIGURE 2.22 Right partial glossectomy.

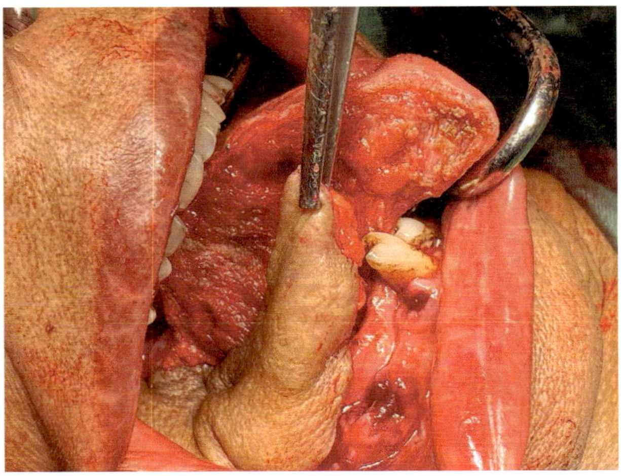

FIGURE 2.23 Setting of platysma flap.

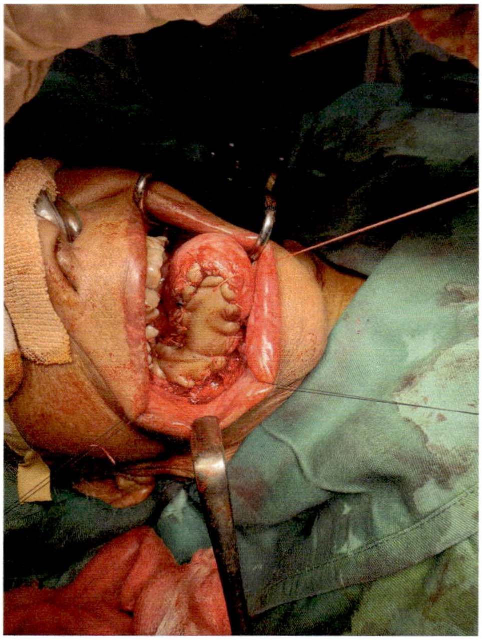

FIGURE 2.24 Flap fully inset.

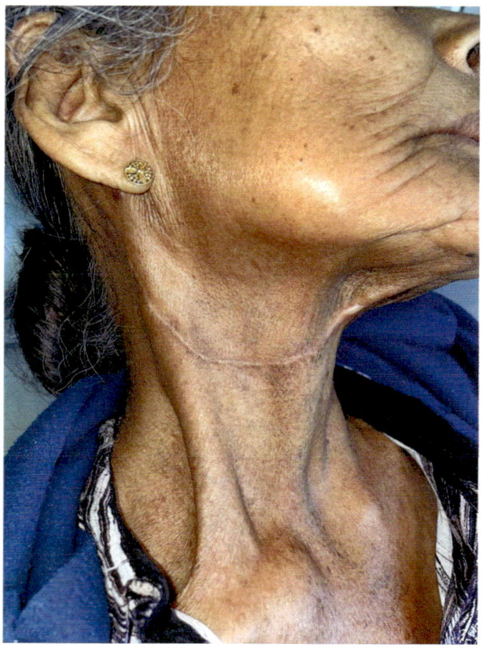

FIGURE 2.25 Post-operative neck wound.

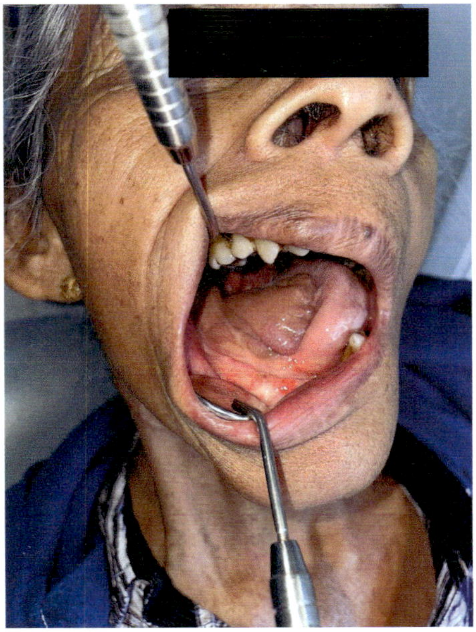

FIGURE 2.26 Post-operative tongue after several months.

Case 2.8

An 83-year-old female who uses a wheelchair presented with a large T3 SCC and underwent a wide local excision. She was not medically fit for neck dissection. The wound was primarily closed (Figures 2.27 and 2.28).

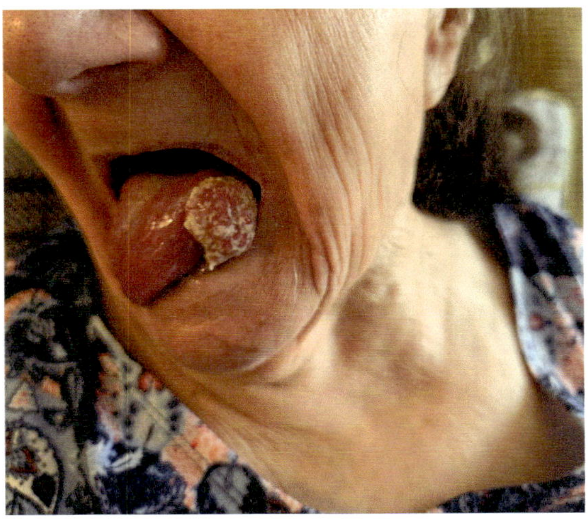

FIGURE 2.27 T2 SCC of the left lateral tongue.

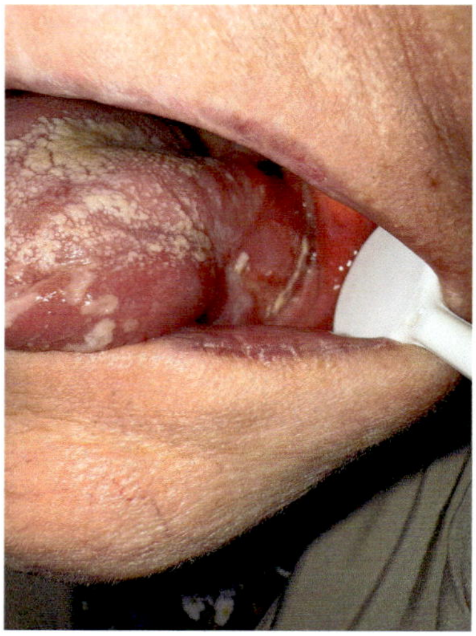

FIGURE 2.28 Three months post-surgery.

Case 2.9

An 80-year-old edentulous female underwent wide local excision of a T2 SCC and an FAMM flap to cover the defect. The donor site was closed with a buccal fat pad. The flap was later divided on its pedicle to create a sulcus and allow her denture to fit (Figures 2.29–2.31).

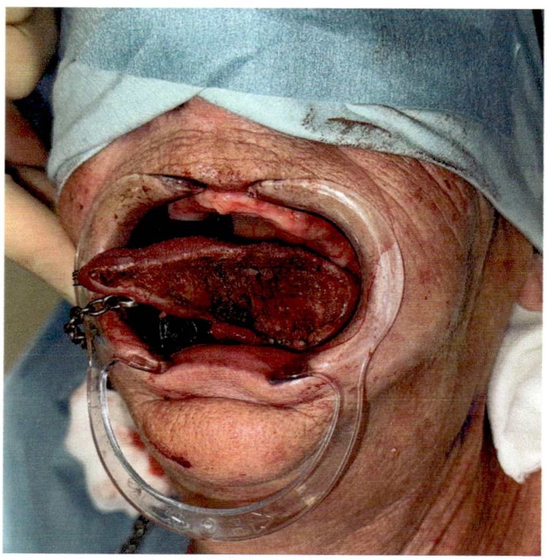

FIGURE 2.29 T2 left tongue SCC following excision

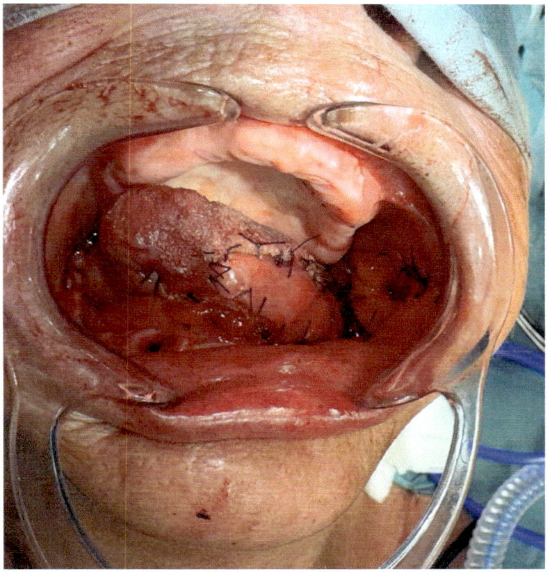

FIGURE 2.30 Left FAMM flap and donor site closure with buccal fat pad.

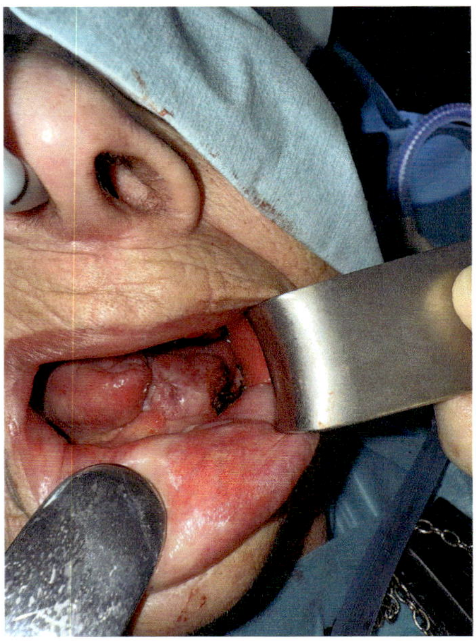

FIGURE 2.31 FAMM flap divided to provide sulcus for dentures.

Cases 2.10, 2.11, 2.12, and 2.13

Various techniques can be used to cover the wound bed to aid healing, reduce bleeding, and improve patient comfort (Figures 2.32–2.39).

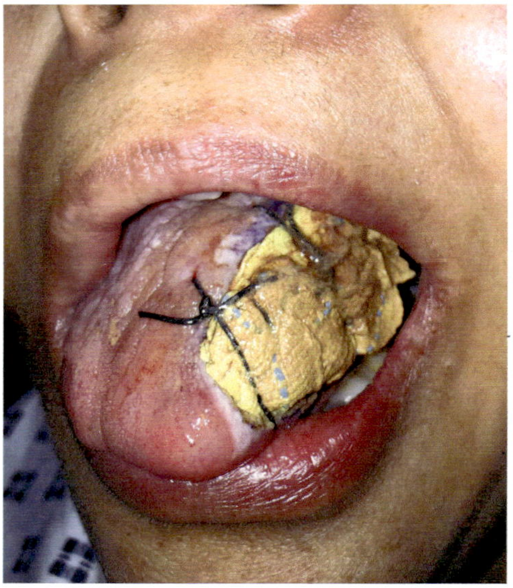

FIGURE 2.32 BIPP sutured in.

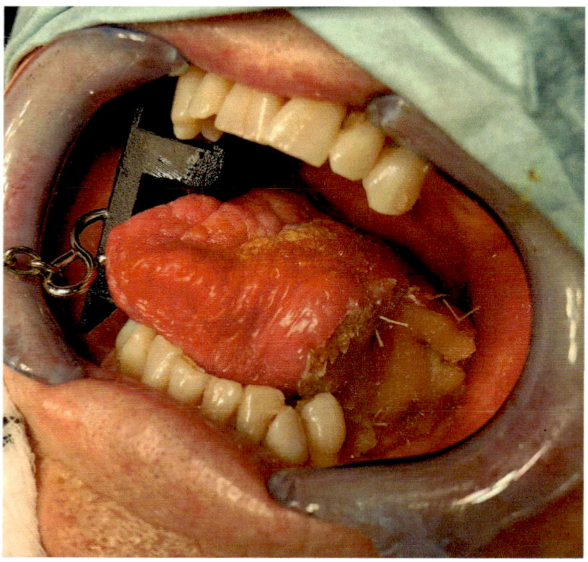

FIGURE 2.33 Well-healed graft in the surgical bed.

Case 2.14

A patient with SCC left lateral tongue, underwent a wide local excision and reconstruction with platysma flap.

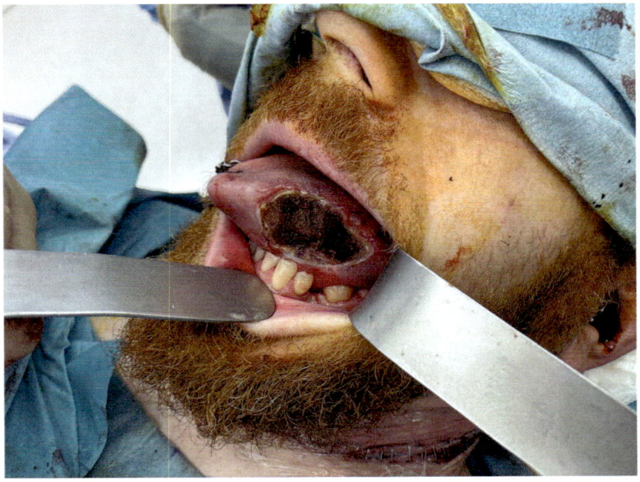

FIGURE 2.34 Wide local excision of T1 SCC.

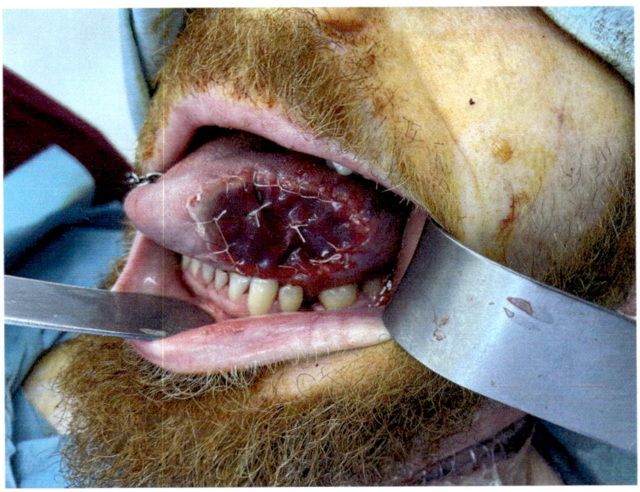

FIGURE 2.35 Synthetic xenograft (integra).

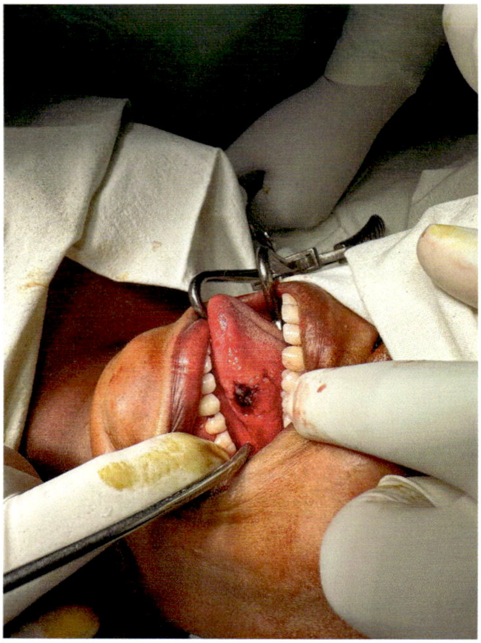

FIGURE 2.36 Left lateral tongue SCC.

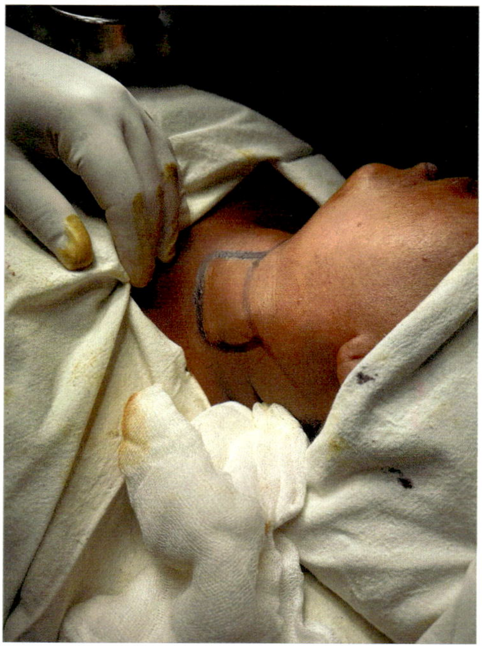

FIGURE 2.37 Left infrahyoid flap outlined.

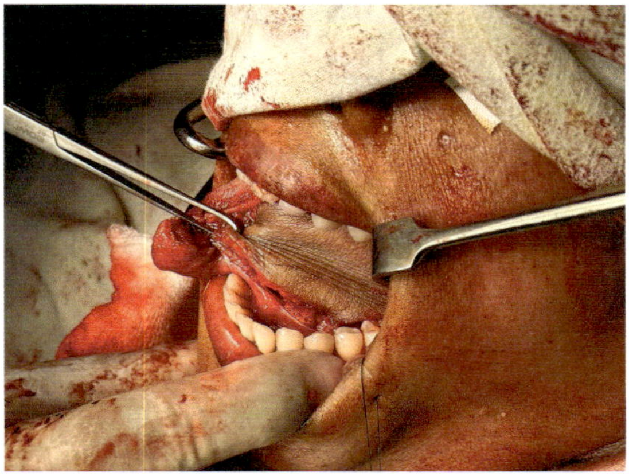

FIGURE 2.38 Flap rotated into oral cavity.

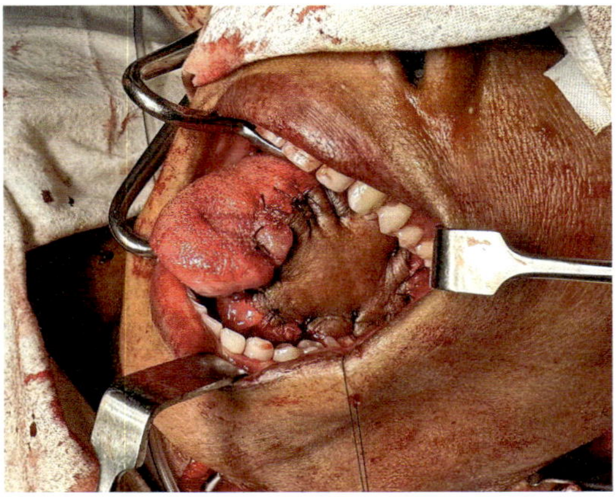

FIGURE 2.39 Flap inset.

DISCUSSION

Oral tongue cancer, typically SCC, is one of the most common malignancies in the oral cavity. It affects the mobile portion of the tongue, making it crucial to manage it appropriately due to the tongue's essential role in speech, mastication, and swallowing. The management of oral tongue cancer involves a multidisciplinary approach, including surgery, radiation therapy, chemotherapy, and reconstruction, with each treatment tailored to the tumor stage, size, and patient-specific factors.

Surgery is the cornerstone for treating oral tongue cancer, particularly in early stages of the disease (T1 and T2 lesions).

CONTROVERSIES IN THE MANAGEMENT OF ORAL TONGUE CANCER

Despite advances in surgical techniques and adjuvant therapies, certain aspects of oral tongue cancer management remain controversial.

Elective Neck Dissection in Early-Stage Disease (T1/T2, N0)

- There is ongoing debate over whether elective neck dissection (END) should be performed in early-stage oral tongue cancers (T1/T2) with clinically negative necks (N0). While the risk of occult metastasis is around 20–30%, some argue that observation with close follow-up is a reasonable approach.
- The role of sentinel node biopsy as a diagnostic tool is starting to be used in many centers, and the authors believe it has a valuable role in some patients.

Surgical Margins

- Defining adequate surgical margins in oral tongue cancer resection remains a topic of debate. A margin of 5 mm or more is generally considered adequate, but some argue that even a close margin can be acceptable with no risk of increase in local recurrence.
- The balance between preserving function and achieving clear margins is a challenge, particularly in tumors close to vital structures like the floor of the mouth.
- The authors believe, due to specimen contracture, vital structures, and several meta-analysis demonstrating no difference in local control, a margin greater than 2.5 mm is adequate.

Adjuvant Radiotherapy in Early-Stage Disease

- The role of adjuvant radiotherapy in patients with early-stage disease but adverse features, such as perineural invasion or lymphovascular invasion, is debated. Some clinicians advocate for the routine use of adjuvant radiation in these cases to reduce the risk of local recurrence.
- The authors all agree that radiation should be reserved for cases with positive margins or nodal metastasis due to the risk of long-term side effects such as xerostomia and osteoradionecrosis.

CHAPTER 3

Lip

KEY POINTS

- **High Visibility and Early Detection**: Lip cancers, particularly on the lower lip, are often detected early due to their prominent location. However, they carry recurrence rates of 5–35% depending on tumor size and location.
- **Distinct Behavior from Oral Cavity Cancers**: Unlike other oral cancers, lip carcinomas behave more like cutaneous carcinomas, with a lower metastasis rate to cervical lymph nodes (5–20%), predominantly involving level I nodes.
- **Surgical and Radiotherapy Options**: Surgery is the primary treatment for lip SCC, but radiotherapy is a viable option for early-stage lesions or for patients unable to undergo surgery. Both approaches offer comparable outcomes in early-stage disease.
- **Reconstruction Challenges**: Achieving functional and aesthetic reconstruction after lip cancer surgery is complex, requiring techniques that preserve oral competence, speech, and appearance, especially for extensive defects.

The lips form the central aesthetic focal points of the lower third of the face, serving pivotal roles in speech articulation, proprioception, and ensuring oral competency for maintaining a seal during the initial phase of swallowing. The arrangement of mucosa, muscle, and skin layers presents notable challenges to reconstructive surgeons. The orbicularis oris muscle is the major circular muscle sphincter of the lips, acting with several radially orientated dilator muscles, which provide antagonism to the

DOI: 10.1201/9781032714585-3

orbicularis. This complex arrangement of muscles allows the stomion to achieve both a wide circular "O" and a narrow slit configuration, which is essential for normal oral function. The anatomical arrangement of the muscles at the commissures is a challenge to recreate, making reconstruction of all but the smallest defects at this site difficult.

The motor nerve supplies to the lip sphincter complex are from the zygomatic, buccal, and mandibular branches of the facial nerve.

The superior and inferior labial arteries provide the lips with a rich blood supply; coupled with this are the numerous points of anastomosis to the contralateral vessels. This permits the extensive mobilization of lip tissue (plus adjacent skin) on a narrow vascular pedicle for the reconstruction of large defects.

A pivotal anatomical reference is the vermilion border, which marks the transition between the skin and the reddish vermilion portion of the lip.

Aesthetic considerations include replicating the vermilion border, recreating the Cupid's bow, and aligning the texture and color of the reconstructed tissue with the surrounding lip.

LOWER LIP DEFECTS

Lower lip defects are secondary to trauma and neoplasm. Achieving oral competence and preventing drooling should be the main aims of reconstruction in these patients. An array of local flaps have been utilized in the reconstruction of such defects.

V-Y or W Wedge Excision

- The defects less than one-third of the lower lip can be reconstructed using a V or W excision.
- The leveling and alignment of the lip vermillion–cutaneous junction is the key step to prevent an obvious flaw in the post-healing period.

Estlander/Abbe–Estlander Flap

- Primarily based on the superior or inferior labial artery for lower and upper lip reconstruction, respectively.
- The commissural defects necessitate the use of the Abbe–Estlander flap, and it usually is a single- stage process.

- On the other hand, the Abbe flap is a two-step process.
- Upper and lower flaps are designed in a similar fashion with an incision camouflaged in the melolabial crease. Rounding off the commissure sometimes requires commissuroplasty.
- Donor site morbidity is more common while using the upper lip due to its relationship with the central lip and nasal subunits.

Staircase or Step Flap

- Primarily used for medial full-thickness defects involving one-third to two-thirds of the lower lip.
- The advantage is the placement of a scar in the mental crease for a better aesthetic outcome.
- Steps are excised in a sequential fashion along with removing the Burow triangle at the end.

Karapandzic Flap

The Karapandzic flap is an ideal example of a circumoral full-thickness rotation advancement flap maintaining the sensory and motor integrity of the lips. The flap is mostly used for full-thickness central lip defects. The preservation of neural and vascular structures is a unique feature of this flap.

Advantages

- Maintains oral sphincter
- No through-and-through incisions preserving neurovascular structures
- Good functionality

Drawbacks

- Microstomia
- Facial scarring
- Distortion of the commissure if the unilateral Karapandzic flap is used

Harvesting Technique

The incisions for the flap start at the base of the pre-existential defect (preferably in the mental crease) through the skin and subcutaneous tissue and travel along the commissure to the melolabial crease up to the ala of the nose. Then blunt dissection is done along the direction of nerves and vessels to stretch the muscle fibers and neurovascular structures. A separate mucosal incision is made 1–2 cm from the edge of the defect, posteriorly facilitating both the flaps to advance toward the midline. Finally, the closure is done in layers.

Webster Bernard Flap

Total lower lip reconstruction is challenging, and local flaps have limitations when it comes to restoration of adequate function, sensation, and height. Many surgeons opt for free flap reconstruction in an ideal situation. Webster modification of the Bernard flap has been considered as one of the options for complete lower lip defect coverage at the expense of a tight lower lip, bulky upper lip, and compromised specialized lip function.

Harvesting Technique

After the lower lip resection, two horizontal incisions are made:

- First, laterally from the commissure.
- Second, laterally from the base of the lower lip defect, dividing the orbicularis but maintaining the buccinator.
- Four Burow triangles situated above and below the lateral flap ends are excised, allowing medial advancement while preventing tight lower lip and excess upper lip.
- Mucosal incisions should be less extensive than skin incisions.
- Care is taken not to injure the branches of the facial nerve
- Tension-free advancement is followed by layered closure.
- In order to create vermillion, mucosal advancement or inferiorly base tongue flap can be used.

Gillies Fan Flap

A Gillies fan flap is characterized by placing a full-thickness incision on the contralateral side of the resection to transfer the entire remaining lip, thus incorporating the oral commissure. Unlike the Karapandzic flap, the Gillies fan flap does not preserve the integrity of neurovascular structures, as the incision is full thickness.

Drawbacks

- Non-sensate flap
- Little muscle function
- Distortion of the commissure requiring commissuroplasty

CLINICAL CASES

Case 3.1

A 42-year-old male diagnosed with SCC of the left lower lip involving labial mucosa and the adjacent skin has been presented to the head and neck clinic. After the diagnostic workup and investigations, the T1 tumor was clinically managed with a wide local excision sparing the left commissure. The remaining defect has been addressed by primary closure. The margins were clear in the final histopathology, and the patient was kept on surveillance (Figures 3.1 and 3.2).

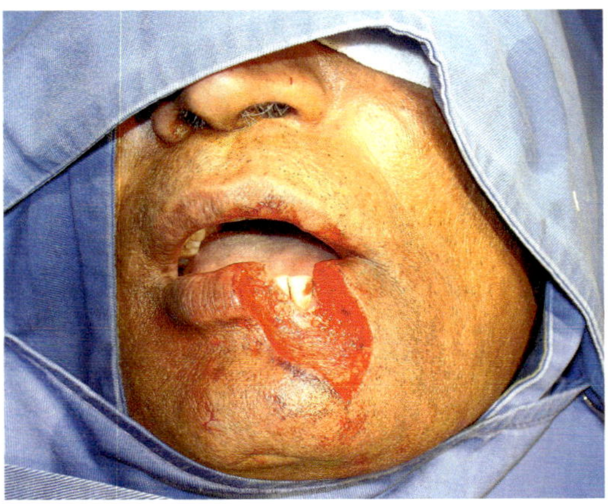

FIGURE 3.1 Ablative defect lower lip.

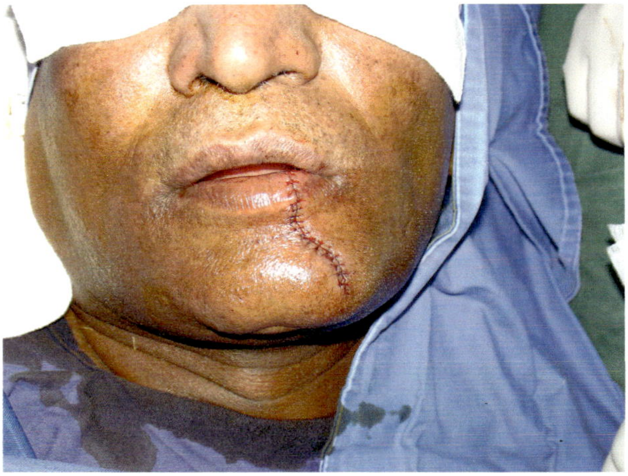

FIGURE 3.2 Primary closure.

Case 3.2

A 50 year old presented with SCC involving the left lower lip commissure. An Abbe–Estlander flap was used to restore oral competence (Figures 3.3–3.7).

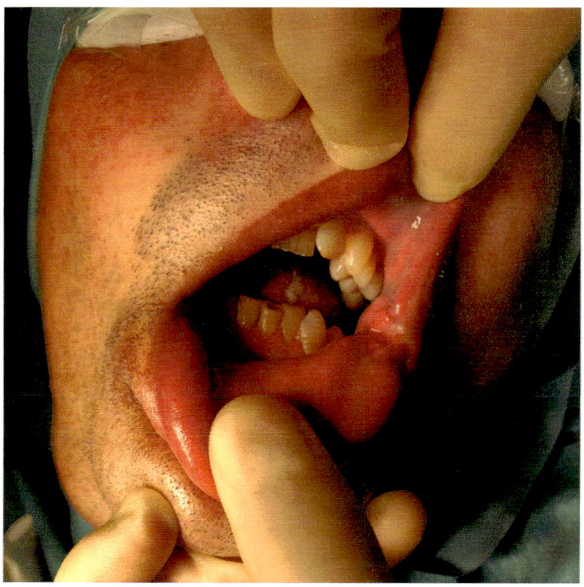

FIGURE 3.3 Lower lip SCC involving commissure.

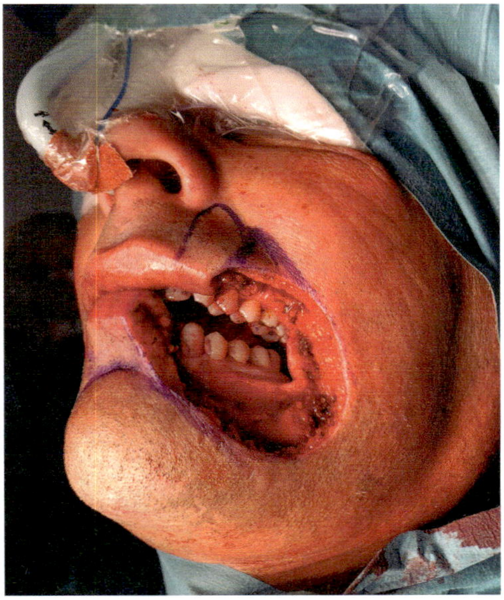

FIGURE 3.4 Defect after excision.

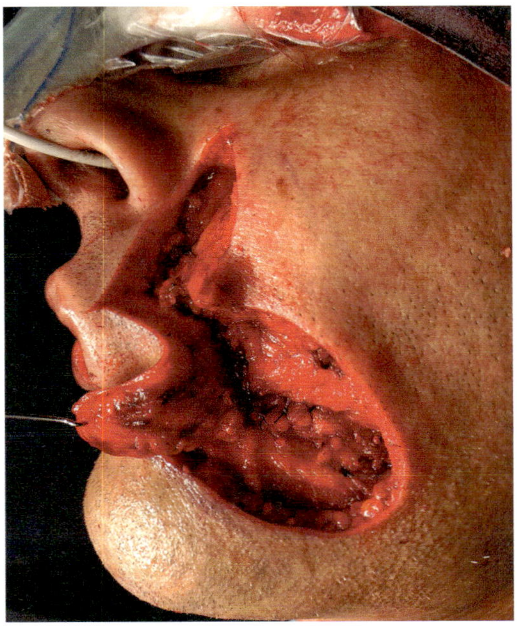

FIGURE 3.5 Full-thickness flap raised.

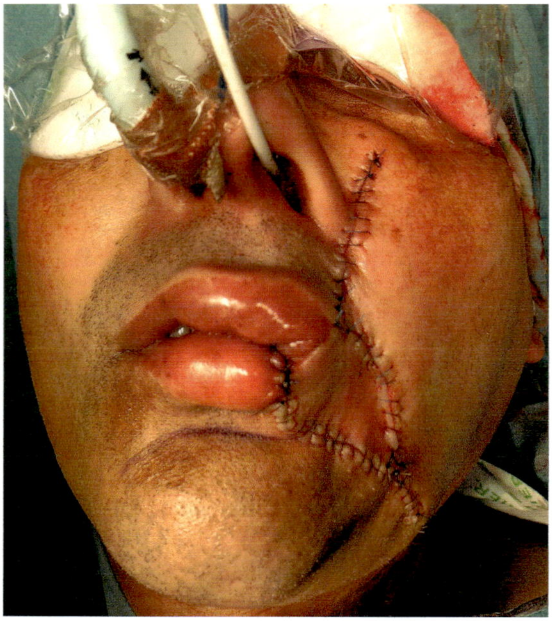

FIGURE 3.6 Flap inset.

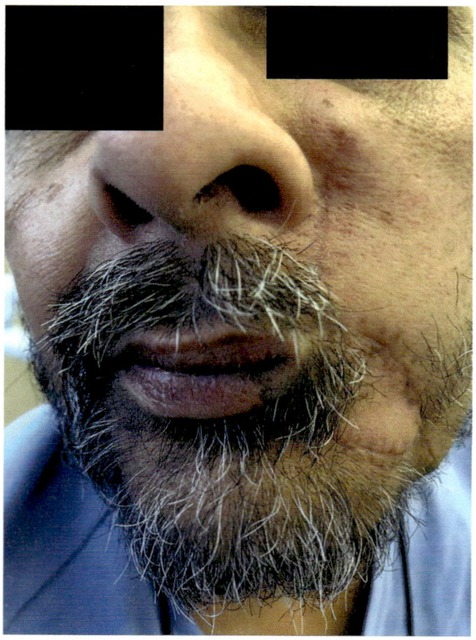

FIGURE 3.7 Three months after surgery.

Case 3.3

A 63-year-old male with a T3N0 lesion has presented to the head and neck unit. After a discussion in MDT, primary resection, bilateral neck dissection, and reconstruction were performed using the Abbe–Estlander and the staircase or step technique of flap advancement. The defect involved two-thirds of the lower lip, including the left commissure, requiring a two-flap approach to achieve the reasonable aesthetic and function outcome (Figures 3.8–3.10).

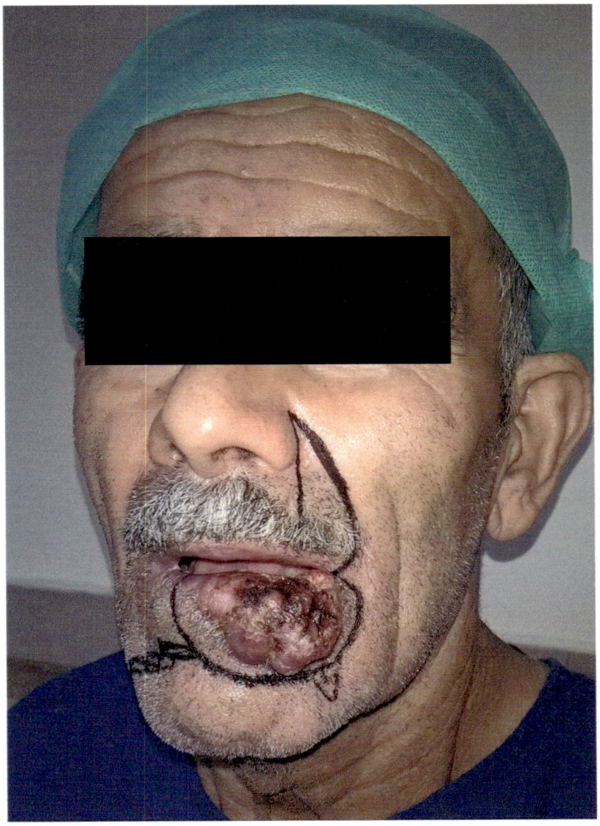

FIGURE 3.8 Lower lip SCC involving two-thirds of the lip, including the commissure.

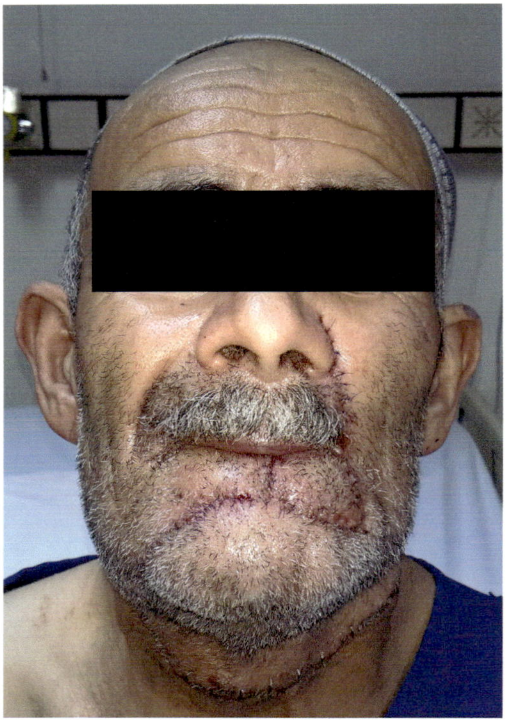

FIGURE 3.9 Reconstruction using Abbe–Estlander and staircase flaps with scars around the mental crease.

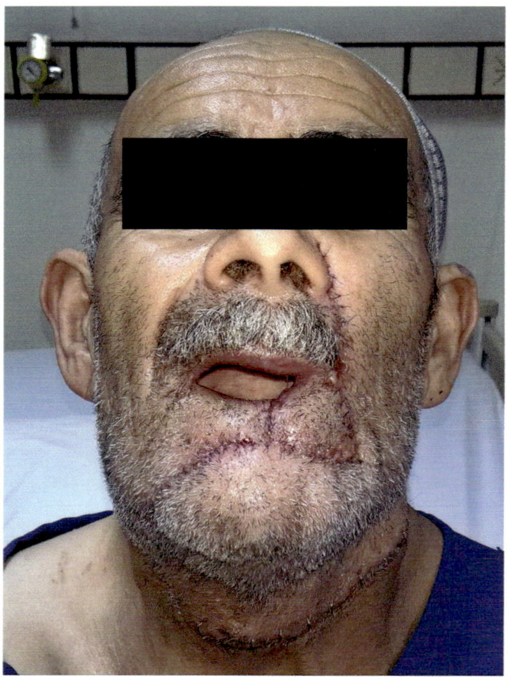

FIGURE 3.10 Post-operative mouth opening.

Case 3.4

A 55-year-old female presented with a one-and-a-half-year history of a lower lip lesion. Clinically, she had a keratotic horn in the background of an erythroplakic indurated lesion with irregular margins, involving 65–70% of the lower lip extending up to the right commissure and right labial sulcus (cT3N0). The biopsy was proven to be positive for well-differentiated SCC. The tumor was excised with adequate margins, and bilateral neck dissection was performed, followed by right-sided nasolabial flap reconstruction. The skin component at the flap base was de-epithelialized to facilitate primary closure of the facial wound (Figures 3.11–3.16).

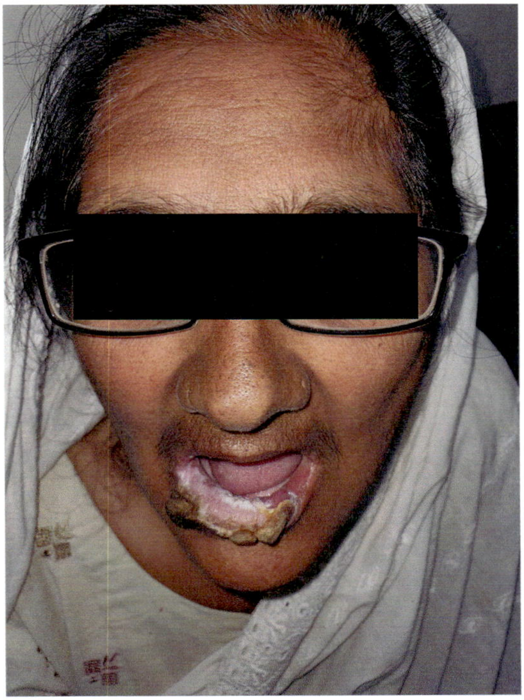

FIGURE 3.11 Lower lip SCC involving more than 65% of the lower lip.

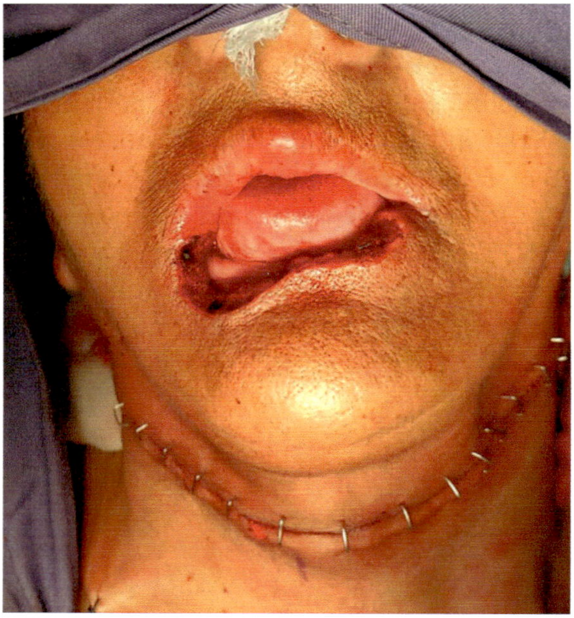

FIGURE 3.12 Defect following excision, involving skin, muscle, and mucosa.

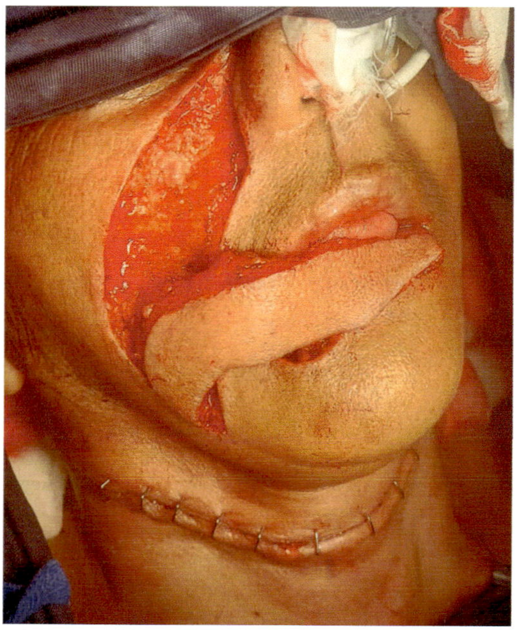

FIGURE 3.13 Right nasolabial flap raised.

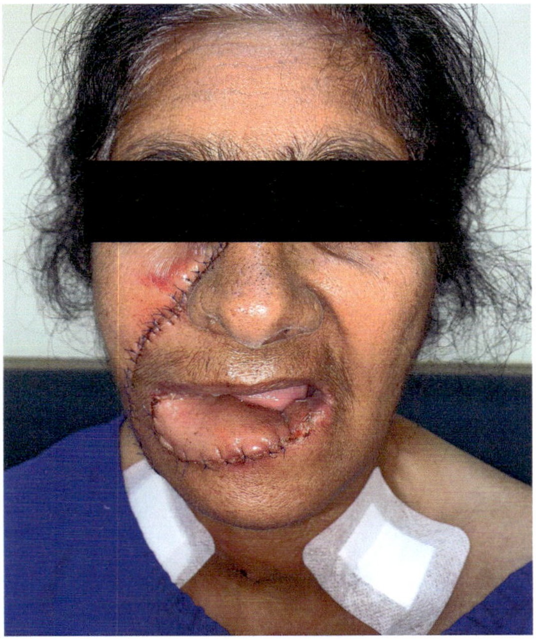

FIGURE 3.14 Three days post-operative.

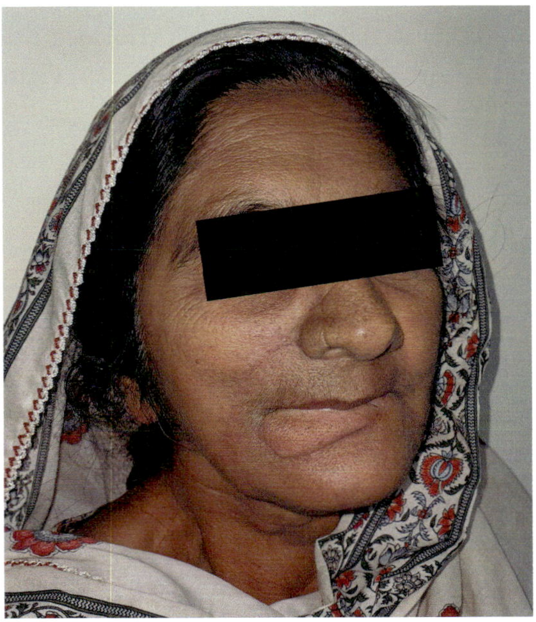

FIGURE 3.15 Scar well-healed and hidden within aesthetic units.

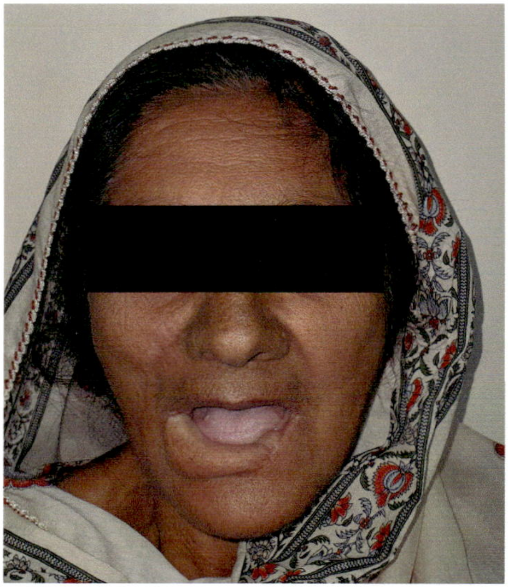

FIGURE 3.16 Good mouth opening.

Case 3.5

A 76-year-old male with a long-standing history of a lower lip lesion involving more than 50% of the lower lip, including the right commissure being diagnosed as SCC. Wide local resection with bilateral neck dissection and immediate reconstruction was performed using a right-side Abbe–Estlander flap and a left-side Karapandzic flap (Figures 3.17–3.22).

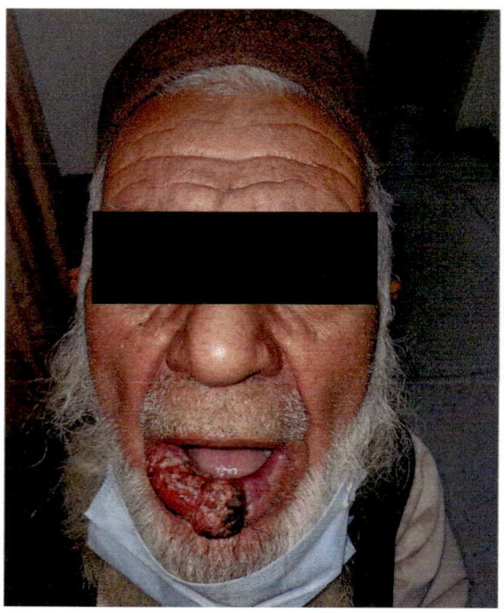

FIGURE 3.17 Right lower lip SCC involving commissure.

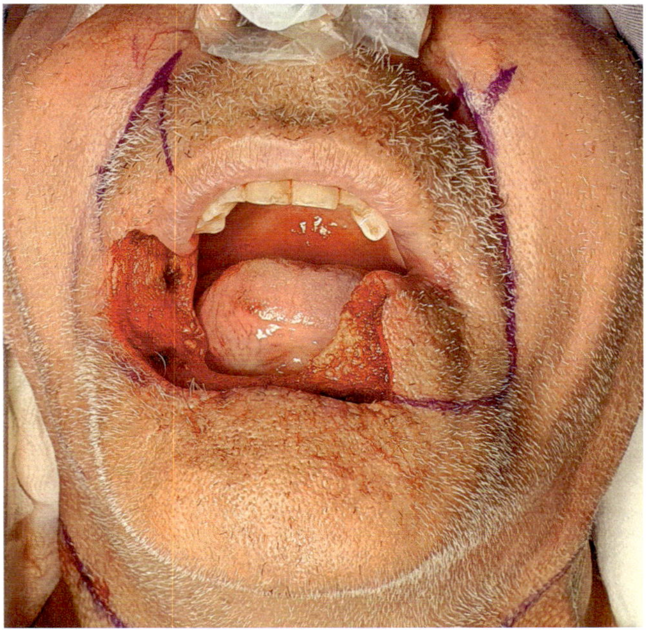

FIGURE 3.18 Defect sparing 25% of the lower lip.

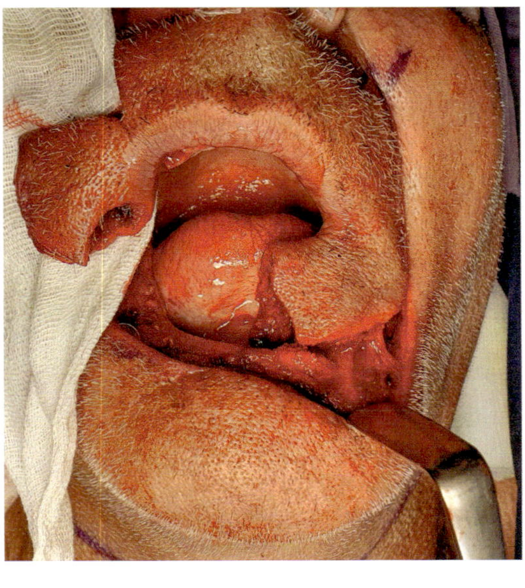

FIGURE 3.19 Right Abbe–Estlander flap and left Karapandzic flap.

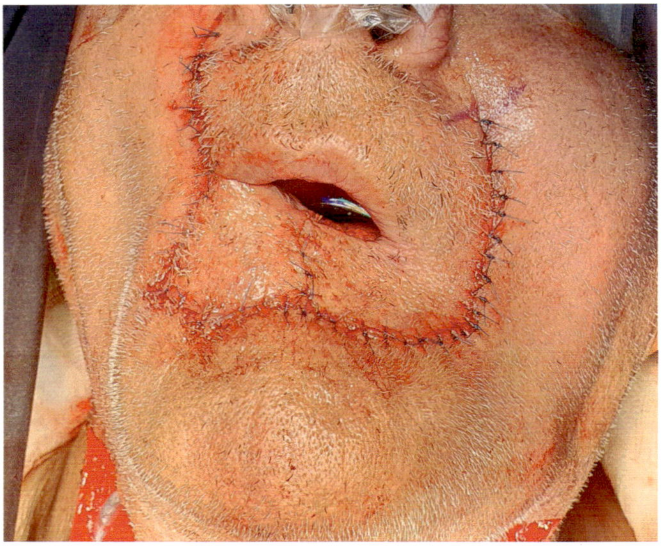

FIGURE 3.20 Immediately post-operative.

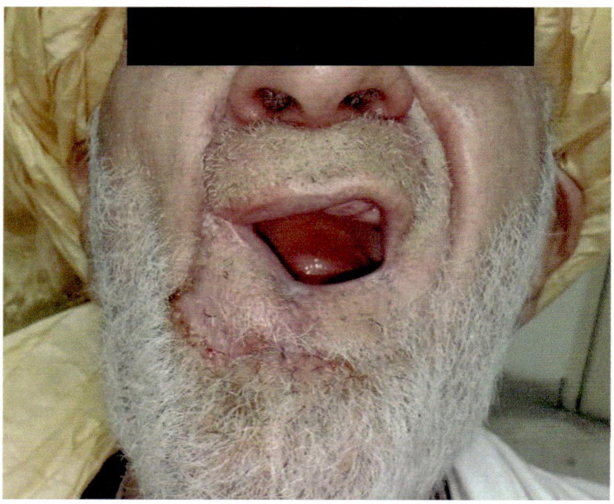

FIGURE 3.21 Four months post-surgery.

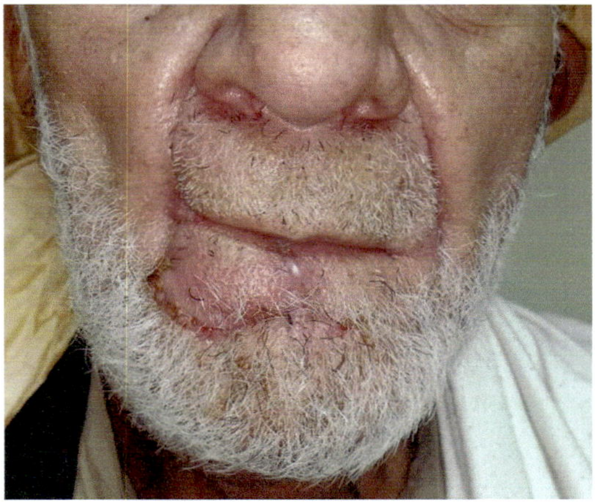

FIGURE 3.22 Good oral seal and scars in the melolabial crease.

Case 3.6

A 50-year-old female with previous radiotherapy and neck dissection developed a new primary commissure. She underwent a wide excision and nasolabial flap (Figures 3.23–3.28).

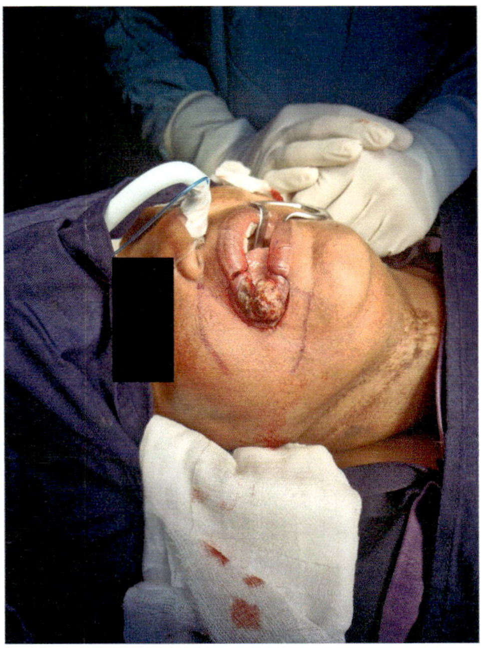

FIGURE 3.23 SCC involving the total lower lip.

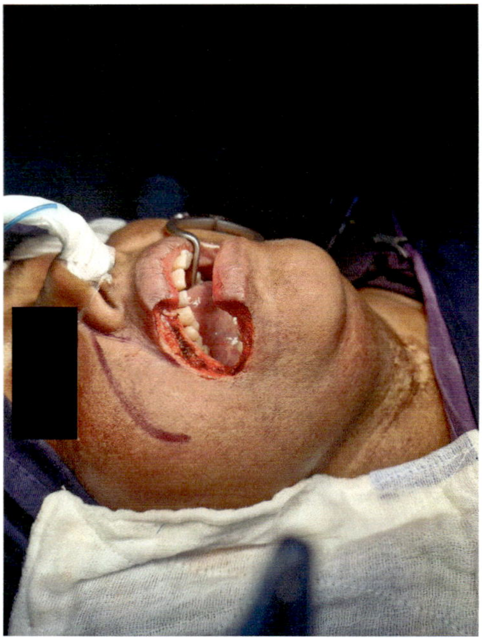

FIGURE 3.24 Defect following resection. Sparing part of the labial mucosa.

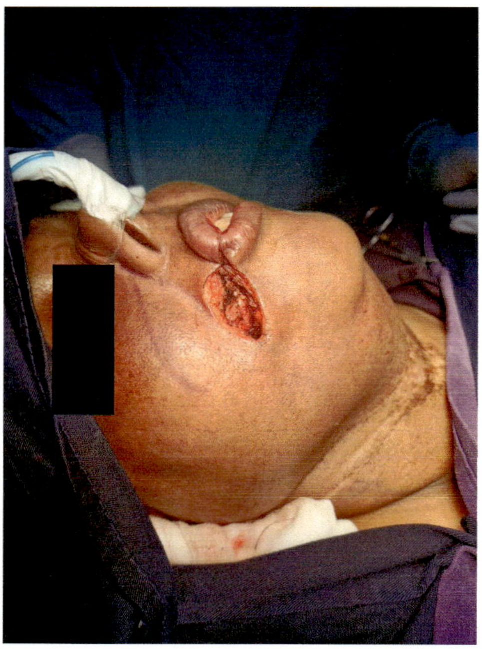

FIGURE 3.25 Bilateral symmetrical Burow triangles are removed.

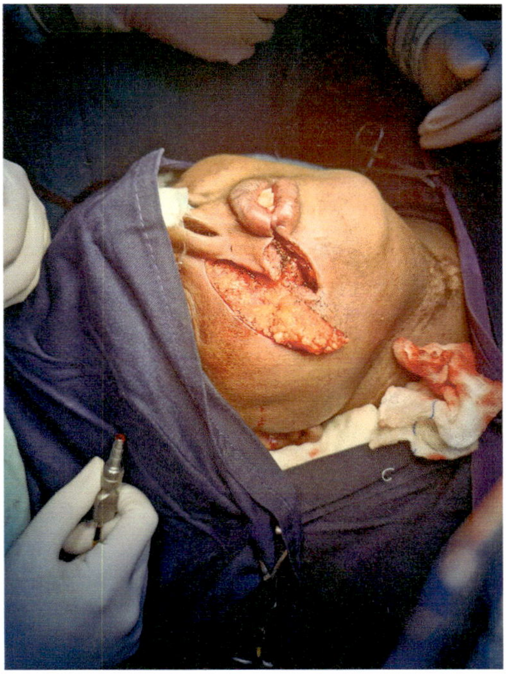

FIGURE 3.26 Horizontal-releasing incisions at the commissure and base of the lip defect bilaterally.

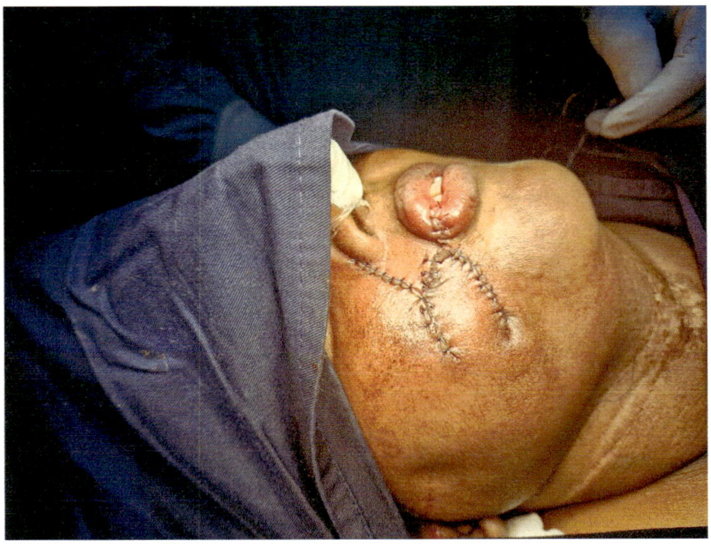

FIGURE 3.27 Four days post-operative.

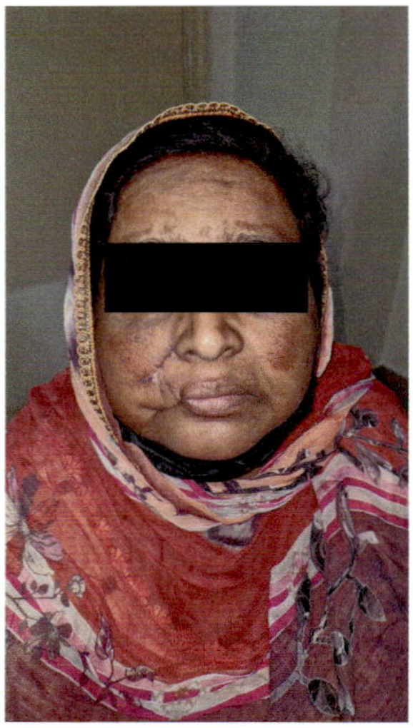

FIGURE 3.28 Good oral seal and lip competency.

Case 3.7

An elderly female presented with biopsy-proven lower lip SCC resected with clear margins. The resection involved the left commissure, resulting in a defect crossing the midline. A left-sided Gillies flap was raised with a standard approach and advanced to cover the defect with a good oral seal (Figures 3.29–3.33).

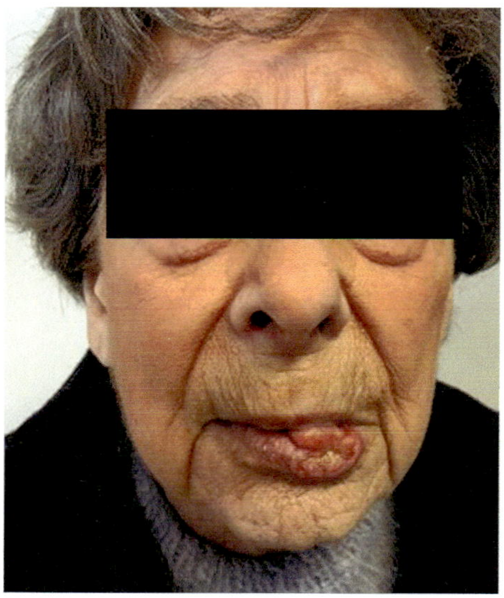

FIGURE 3.29 Lower lip SCC sparing commissure.

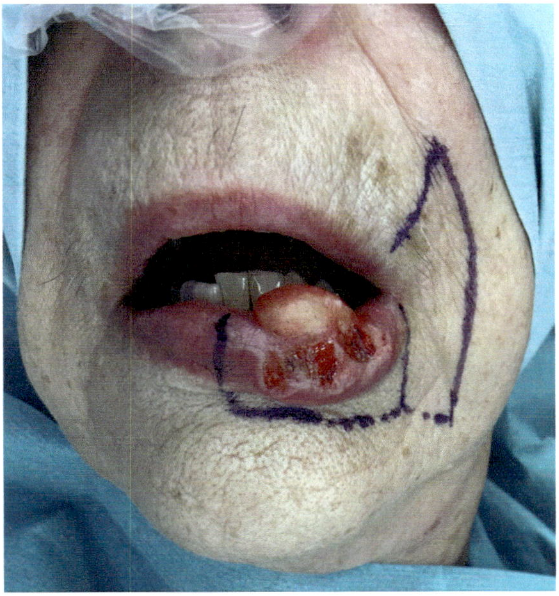

FIGURE 3.30 Ipsilateral Gillies fan flap.

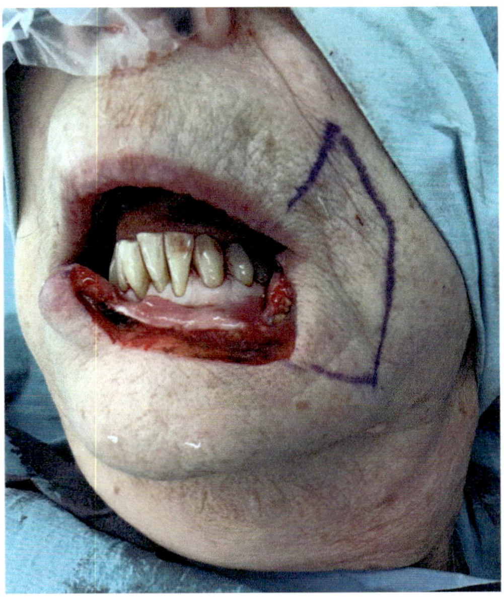

FIGURE 3.31 Defect post-resection sparing right commissure.

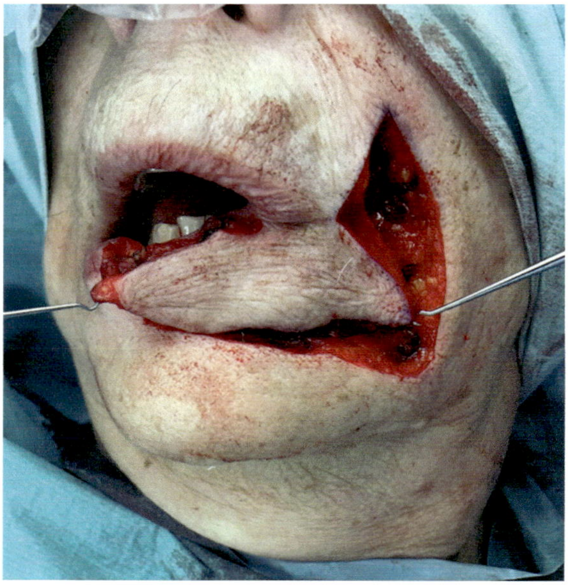

FIGURE 3.32 Full-thickness flap raised and rotated for medial advancement.

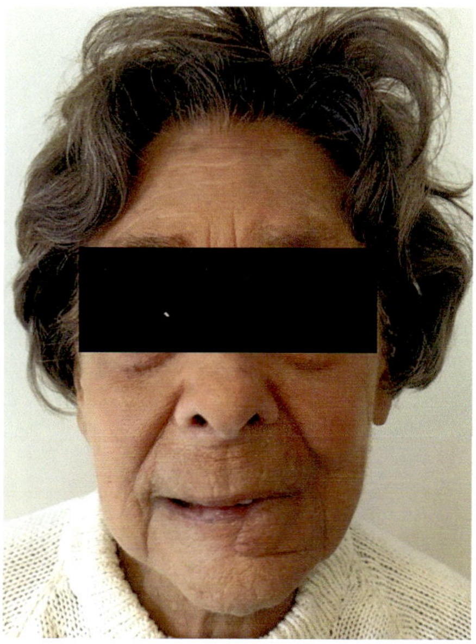

FIGURE 3.33 A well-healed wound and good oral seal.

Case 3.8

A middle-aged female presented with a biopsy of proven lower lip SCC resected with clear margins. The resection was in the midline. A Karapandzic flap was raised with a standard approach and advanced to cover the defect with a good oral seal (Figures 3.34–3.38).

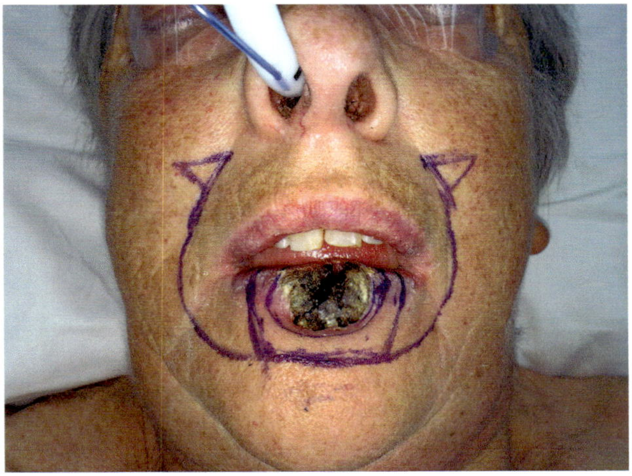

FIGURE 3.34 Lower lip SCC midline with flap markings.

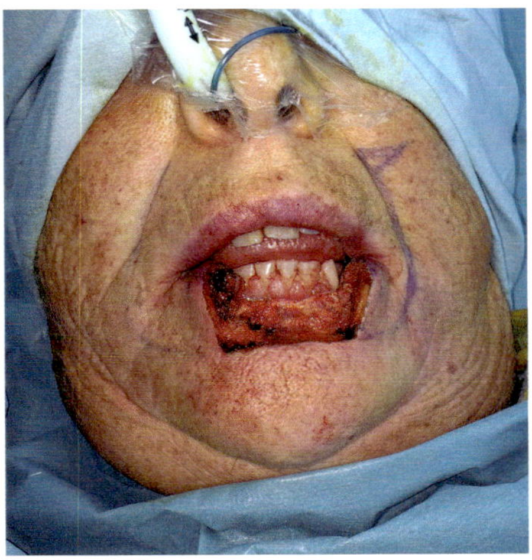

FIGURE 3.35 The defect post-resection.

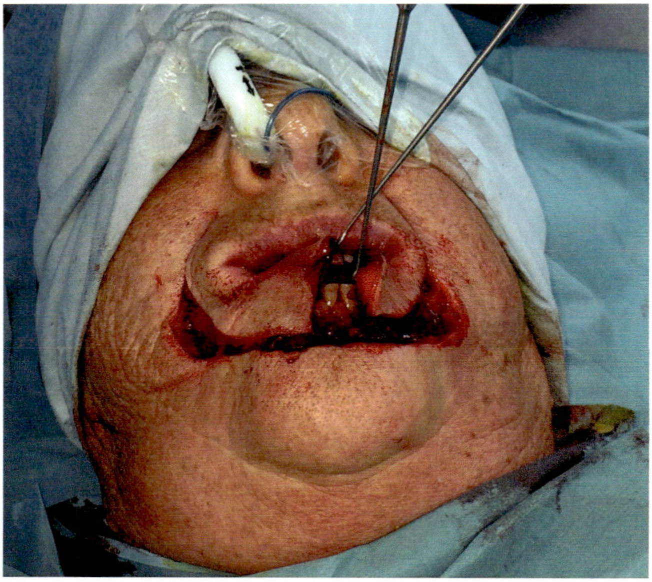

FIGURE 3.36 Full flap raised.

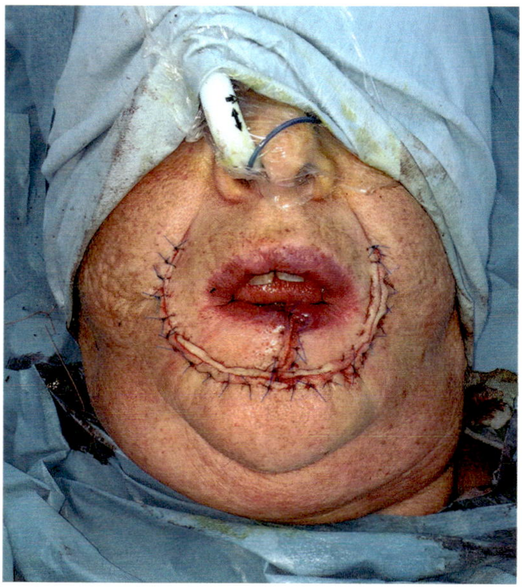

FIGURE 3.37 Flap closed in three layers.

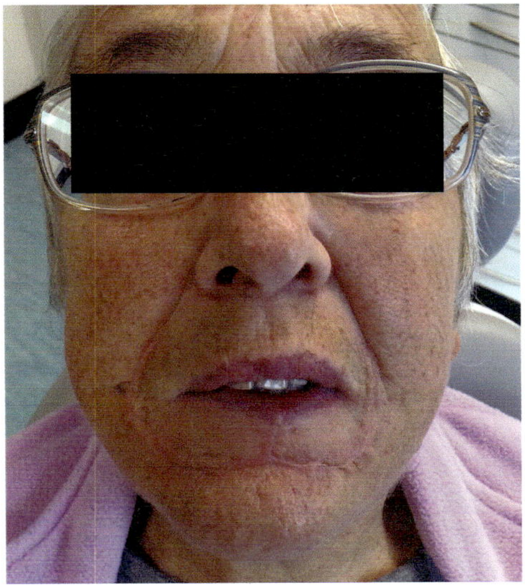

FIGURE 3.38 Three months post-operative with good oral seal and function.

Case 3.9

SCC lower lip underwent wide local excision and stepladder reconstruction with (Figures 3.39–3.41).

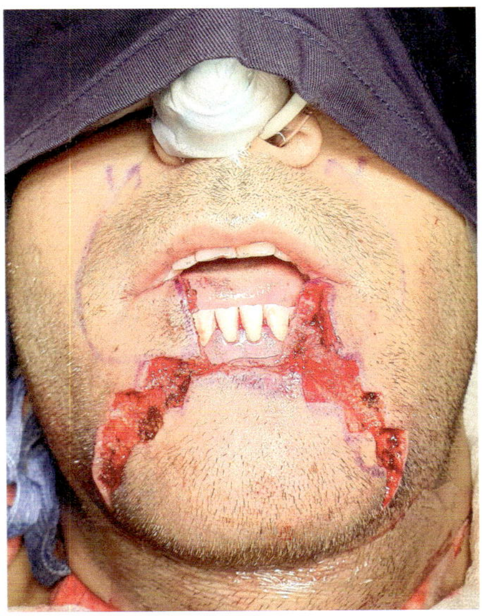

FIGURE 3.39 Lower lip SCC, staircase flap.

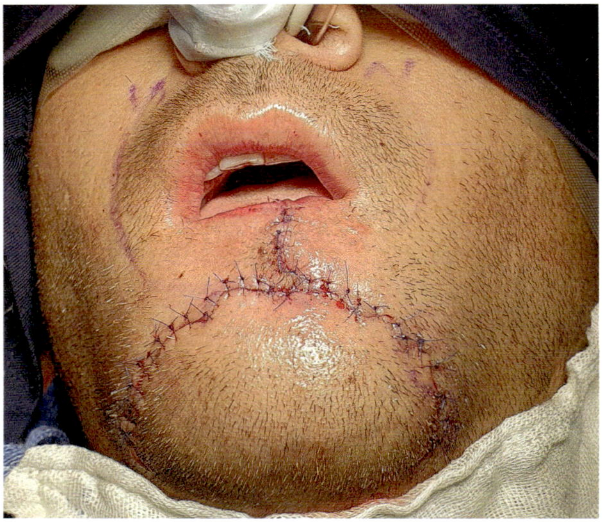

FIGURE 3.40 Immediately post-operative.

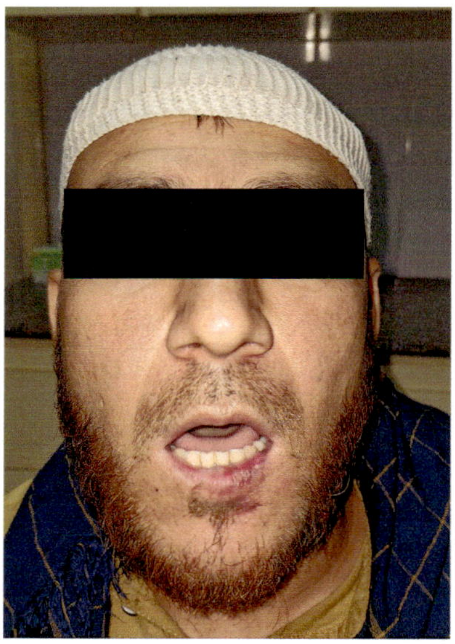

FIGURE 3.41 Three months post-operative.

Case 3.10

An 18 year old with lip SCC midline initially underwent a stepladder reconstruction. The wound became infected and a revision with a bilateral Karapandzic flap was used (Figures 3.42–3.45).

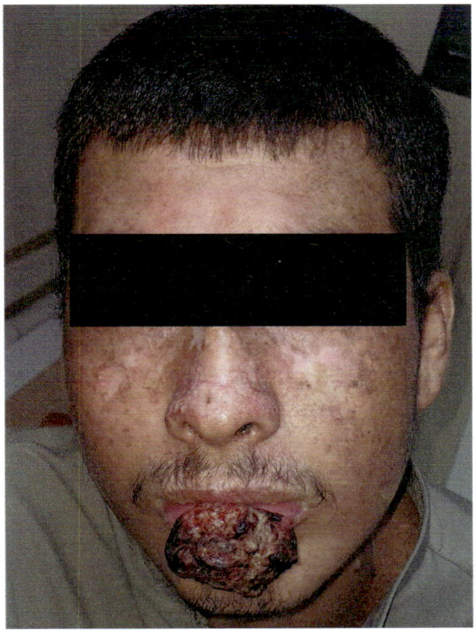

FIGURE 3.42 SCC in the middle of the lower lip.

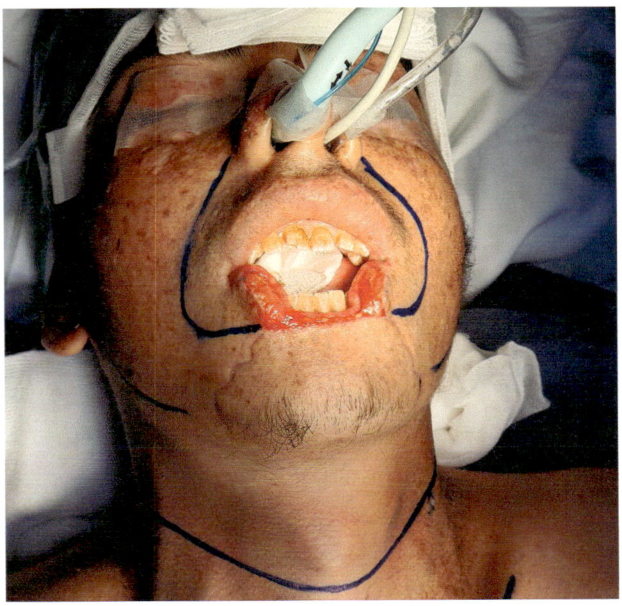

FIGURE 3.43 The patient had a previous stepladder reconstruction that became infected. A bilateral Karapandzic flap was used.

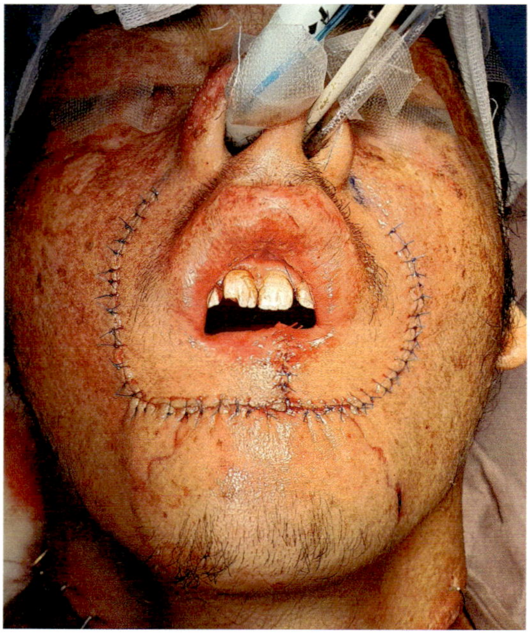

FIGURE 3.44 The flap was sutured.

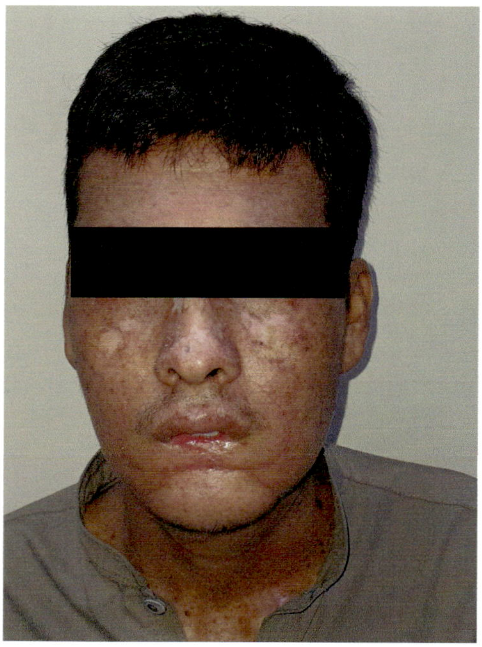

FIGURE 3.45 A few weeks post-operative, well-healed.

UPPER LIP DEFECTS

The upper lip has a midline philtrum and two lateral units comprising philtrum ridges, the Cupid's bow, melolabial/nasolabial folds, and the vermilion border. Defects involving less than 25% of the upper lip are usually addressed by primary closure while those involving over 25% of the upper lip usually require either a single flap or a combination of flaps.

Case 3.11

A 58-year-old male presented with midline upper lip tumor involving the mucocutaneous junction and philtrum ridges, creating a 3.5 × 3 cm defect. To mobilize the alar-sulcus tissue inward toward the defect, skin ellipse was excised and tissue was advanced to cover the defect (Figures 3.46–3.49).

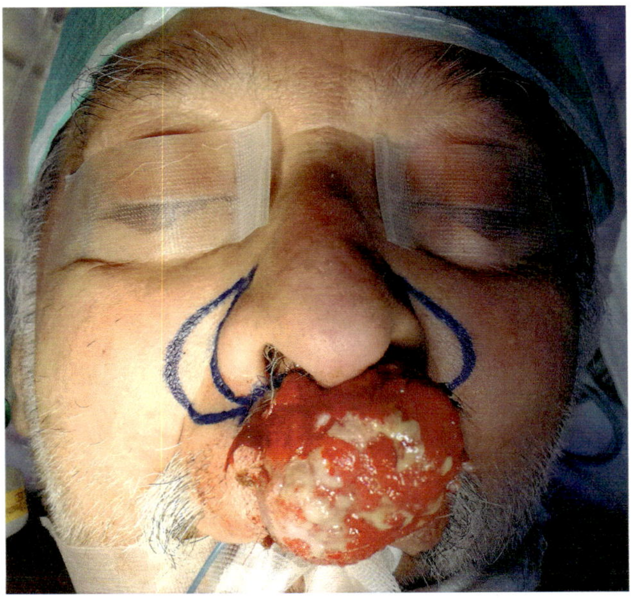

FIGURE 3.46 Upper lip midline, SCC involving the philtrum.

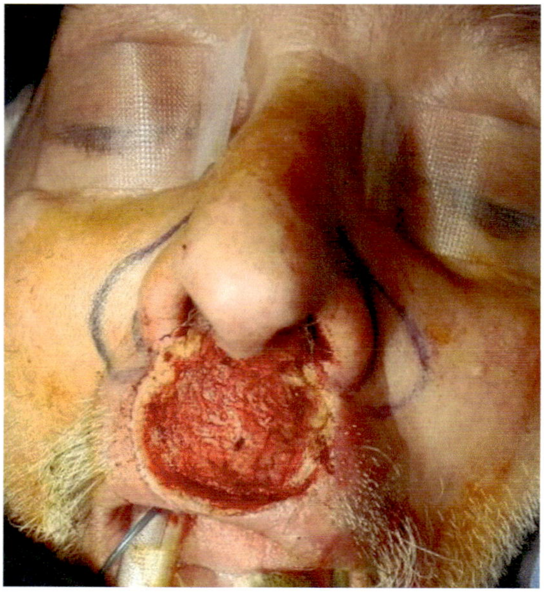

FIGURE 3.47 The defect post-resection with ellipse marked for excision.

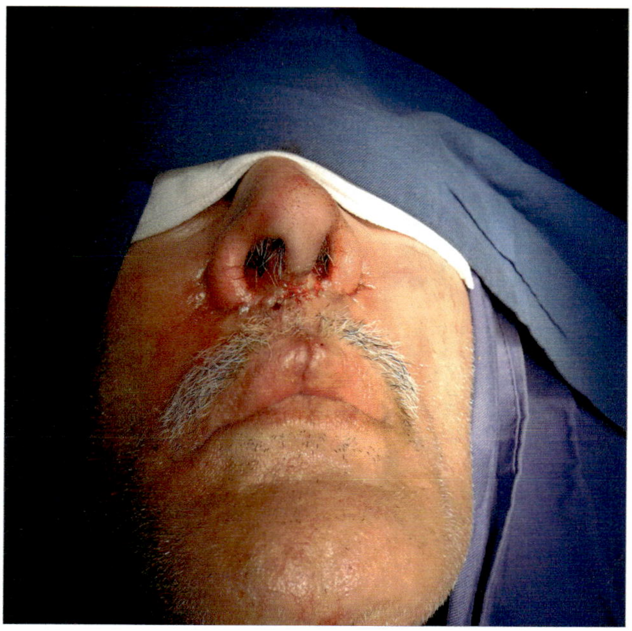

FIGURE 3.48 Five days post-operative.

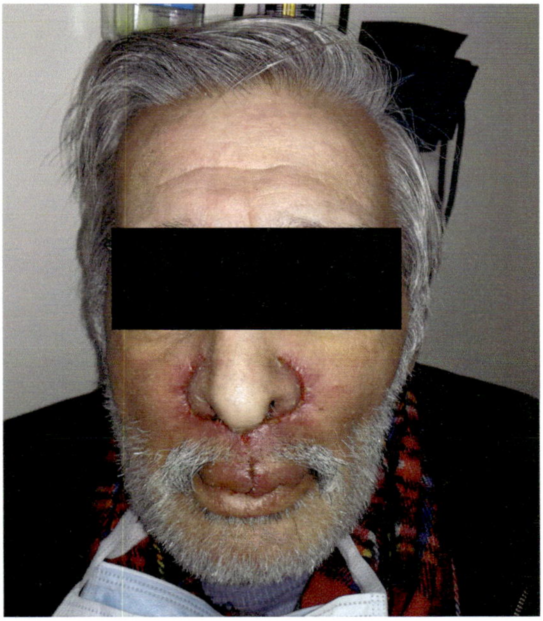

FIGURE 3.49 A well-healed wound with good approximation in the midline.

Case 3.12

A 62-year-old tobacco pipe (hookah) user presented with a history of an upper lip lesion (the biopsy proved it to be basosquamous carcinoma) that started 10 years ago and gradually increased in size so that it has literally involved the entire upper lip, with extension into the left nasolabial crease. Occasional bleeding was one of the recent findings. Wide local resection of the upper lip was done with adequate margins, and reconstruction was performed using paramedian forehead flap reconstruction. The flap stayed congested for a week with gradual improvement in 2 weeks. Flap division was performed at the third week (Figures 3.50–3.53).

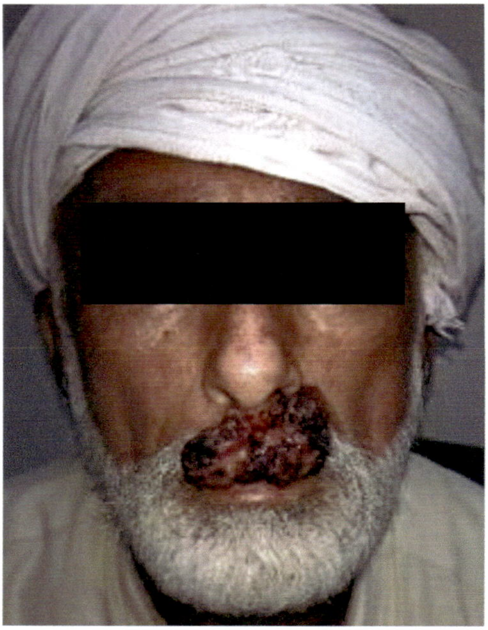

FIGURE 3.50 Extensive upper lip tumor with left nasolabial extension.

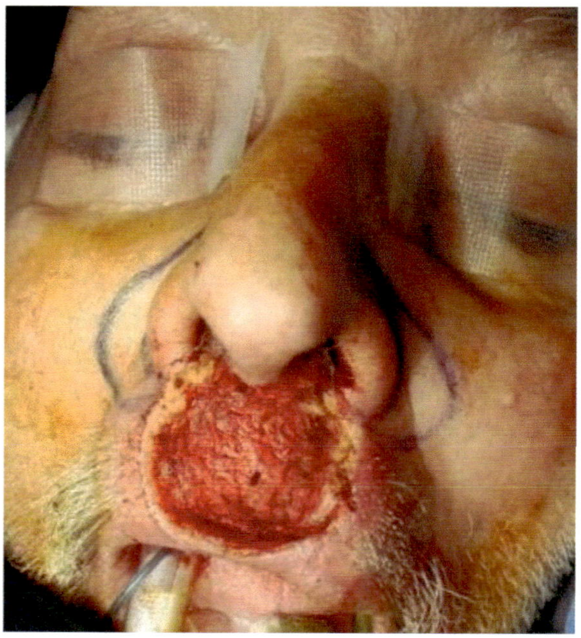

FIGURE 3.51 Wide excision of the primary tumor.

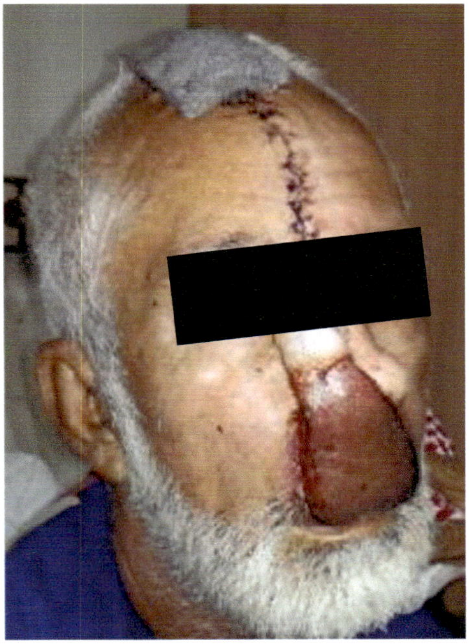

FIGURE 3.52 Congested flap on the third day.

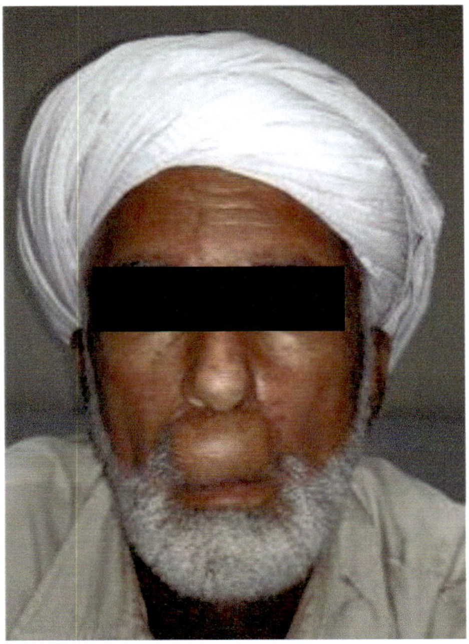

FIGURE 3.53 Well-healed wound after flap division 28 days later.

Case 3.13

A 67-year-old male has a long-standing upper lip BCC located precisely in upper lip. The tumor was excised with adequate margins, and reconstruction was done using an inferior pedicle island flap (Figures 3.54–3.57).

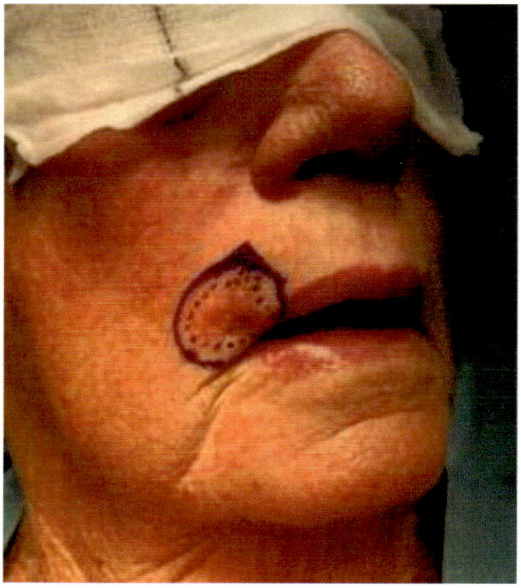

FIGURE 3.54 Lesion of the upper lip.

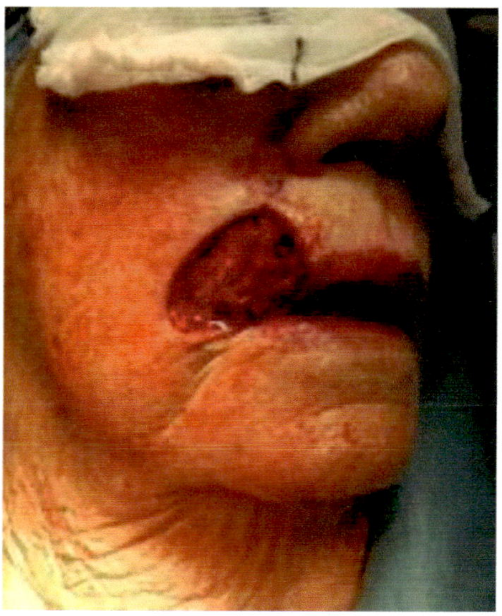

FIGURE 3.55 Resected tumor.

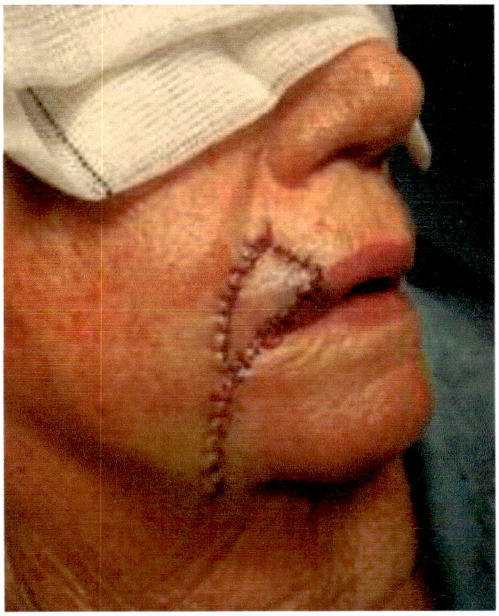

FIGURE 3.56 Pedicled island flap.

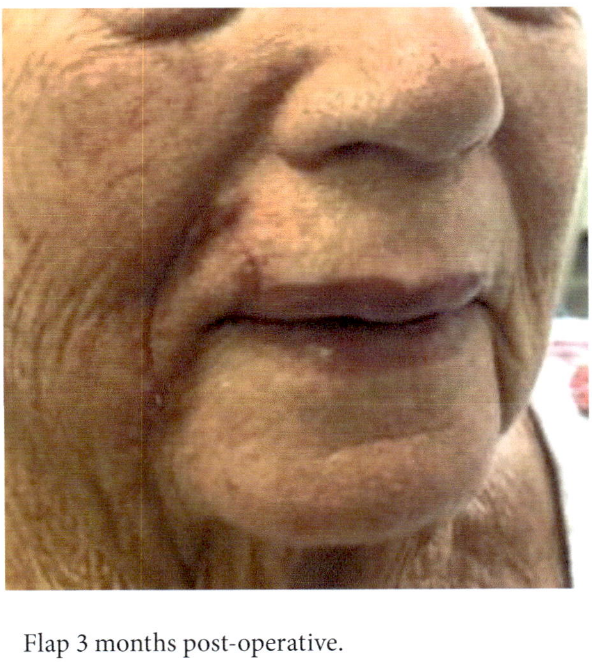

FIGURE 3.57 Flap 3 months post-operative.

Case 3.14

A 60 year old with a long-standing *Candida* infection commissure underwent wide local excision and primary closure (final pathology SCC) (Figures 3.58–3.61).

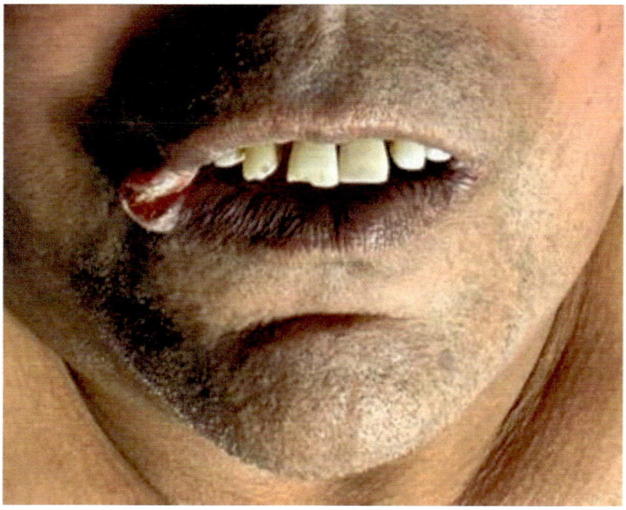

FIGURE 3.58 SCC right commissure.

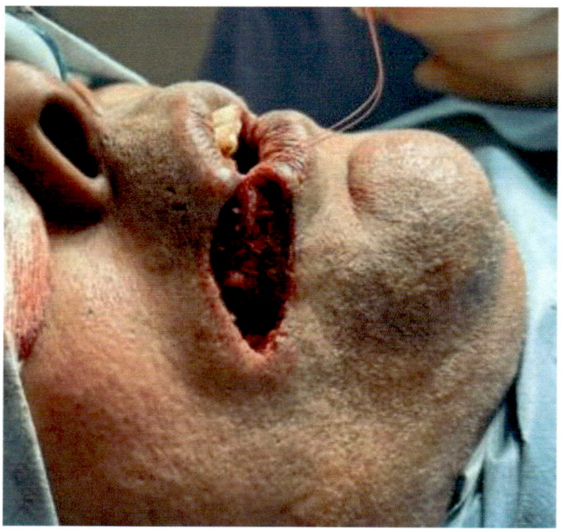

FIGURE 3.59 Three-layer closure.

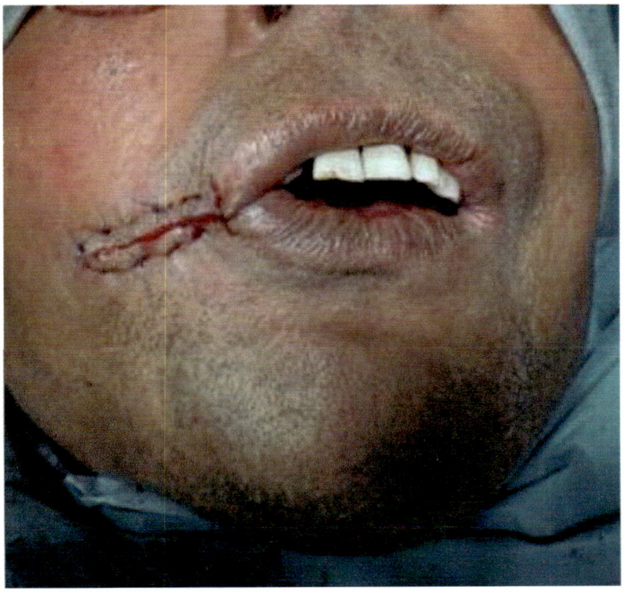

FIGURE 3.60 Primary closure of skin.

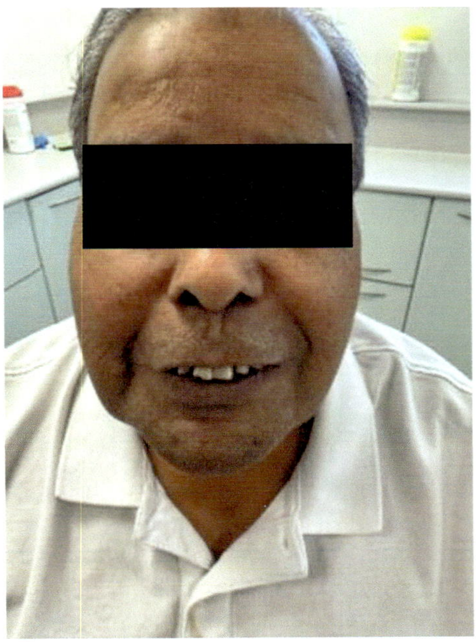

FIGURE 3.61 Six months post-operative.

Case 3.15

An elderly gentleman with SCC of the right upper lip underwent wide local excision and reconstruction with a submental flap (Figures 3.62–3.66).

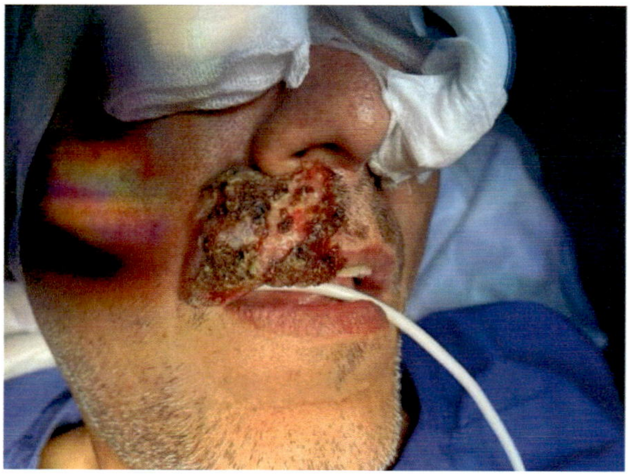

FIGURE 3.62 SCC of the right upper lip.

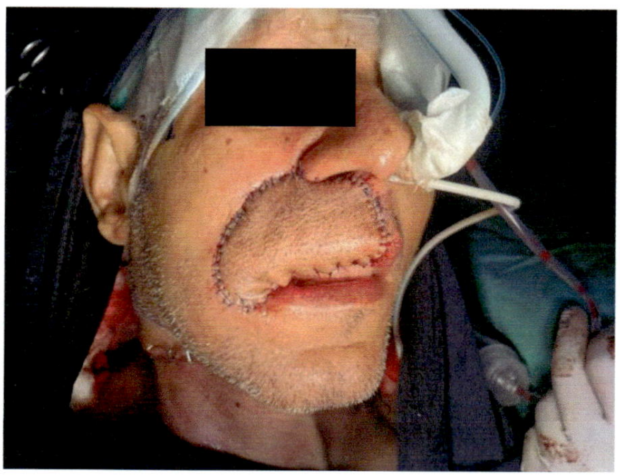

FIGURE 3.63 Immediate post-operative reconstruction with a submental flap.

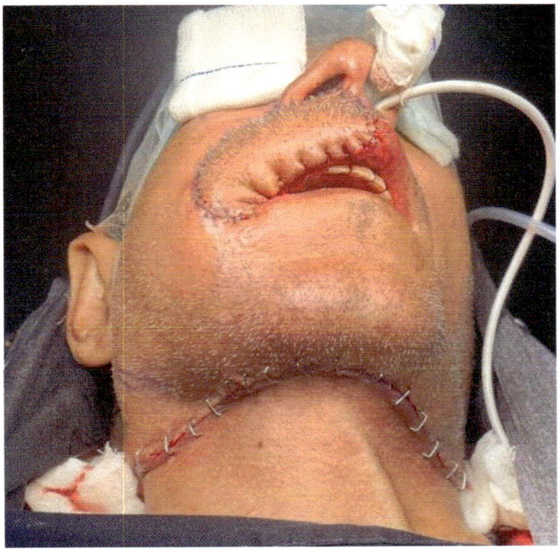

FIGURE 3.64 Neck wound closure.

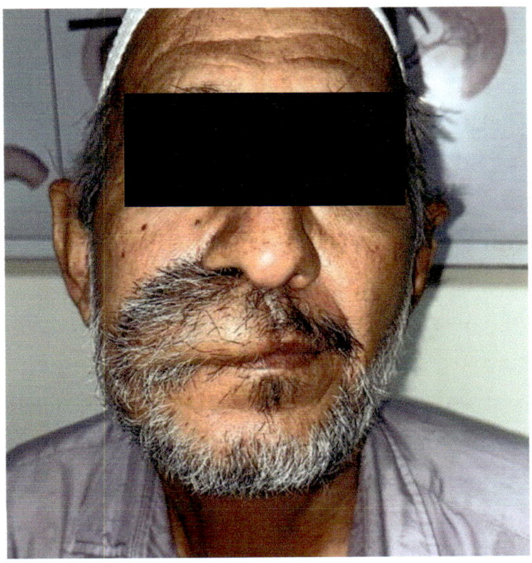

FIGURE 3.65 Three months post-operative.

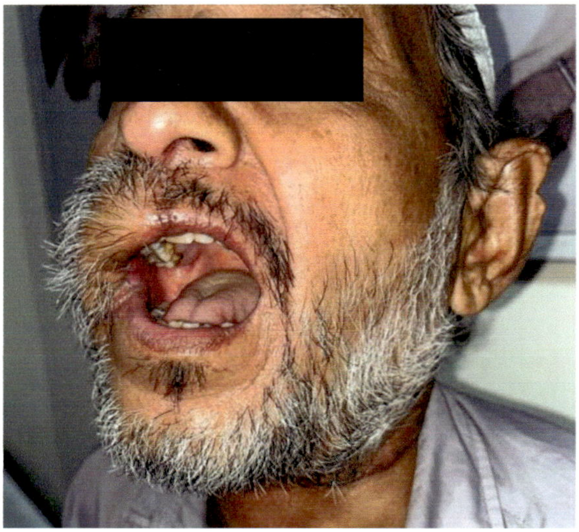

FIGURE 3.66 Three months post-operative, lateral view.

DISCUSSION

Carcinoma of the lip accounts for 25% of oral carcinomas; 82% of lip carcinomas develop on the lower lip, 10% at the upper lip, and 8% at the lateral commissure. Given the high visibility of the lip, most lip carcinomas are detected early. Recurrence rates range from 5% to 35% and are dependent on tumor size, location, and previous treatment.

The behavior of lip carcinomas is distinct from carcinomas of the oral cavity and is primarily managed as a cutaneous carcinoma. The incidence of lip carcinoma metastasis to cervical lymph nodes is 5–20%, with level I involvement being most common. Prophylactic neck dissection is not recommended for early-stage disease; ultrasound of the draining lymph nodes is appropriate for surveillance of the clinically negative neck.

Surgery is regarded as the main treatment modality; radiotherapy should be considered to preserve function and cosmesis, for inoperable tumors, in instances with multiple lesions, and in the post-operative setting for adjuvant management of high-risk features and lymph node involvement. Primary radical radiotherapy and surgery are equal treatment options for early-stage T1–T2 carcinoma, where both achieve good local control. Synchronous dysplasia is evident in half of lip squamous cell carcinomas, with synchronous SCC seen in 5%; presence of synchronous carcinomas can make decision-making more challenging in this patient population.

Primary radical radiotherapy can be particularly useful for elderly patients who may not be suitable for radical surgery due to medical co-morbidities. Adjuvant radiotherapy improves outcomes following primary surgery; case studies report improved recurrence-free survival outcomes (51% cf 92%, $p = 0.008$) in high-risk carcinoma with the addition of post-operative radiotherapy.

Adjuvant radiotherapy should be considered post-operatively for:

- pT3–T4 disease
- Residual disease after surgery
- Close or positive pathological margin (<1 mm)
- Perineural and/or lymphovascular space invasion

For high-risk lip carcinomas, selected institutions deliver 50 Gy elective lymph node irradiation to the first-echelon lymph nodes as an alternative to prophylactic neck dissection; with this approach, the rate of isolated recurrence within electively irradiated lymph nodes is 2.8%. Randomized data are not available, and elective nodal irradiation is not currently considered as the standard of care, but it may be considered on a case-by-case basis for high-risk primary lip carcinomas.

CHAPTER 4

Upper Alveolus, Hard Palate, and Lower Alveolus

KEY POINTS

- **Functional and Aesthetic Challenges**: Defects in the alveolus and palate compromise speech, swallowing, and oral competence, necessitating tailored reconstruction strategies to restore these functions while addressing aesthetic concerns.
- **Reconstruction Options**: Choices range from secondary intention healing for small defects to advanced techniques like nasolabial, palatal island, or temporalis muscle flaps for larger, complex defects. The choice depends on defect size, location, and patient-specific factors.
- **Prosthetic Rehabilitation**: Maxillary obturators are commonly used to create an oro-nasal seal for functional restoration, avoiding nasal speech and achieving oral continence in dentate patients, but they come with challenges such as hygiene maintenance and stability.
- **Considerations in Planning**: Factors such as comorbidities, prior surgeries, radiation, and the quality of residual bone are critical in determining whether bone-containing flaps or soft tissue-only solutions are required.

DOI: 10.1201/9781032714585-4

The upper alveolus and hard palate form the partition between oral and nasal cavities. They also comprise the floor of the maxillary sinus and nasal cavity. The loss of alveolar ridge bone and soft tissue has implications such as compromise in speech, articulation, and oral competence.

The factors to be considered before reconstruction are:

- Comorbidity
- BMI
- Mental status
- Size and location
- Desire for dentition
- Prior surgery
- Previous radiation
- Current dentition status

While planning to reconstruct these defects, one must consider the importance of gingivolabial, gingivobuccal, and lateral tongue space or floor of the mouth. The presence of excessive flap bulk, scarring, or blunting of these key areas can result in disturbance of speech, swallowing, and improper denture adjustment, requiring revision surgeries or vestibuloplasty/commissuroplasty.

Bony and soft tissue defects following tumor resection have different reconstructive objectives requiring simple as well as complex surgical planning. The amount, location, quality of residual bone, dentition, and denture-bearing alveolar arch determine whether a bone containing a flap is required or not.

The use of maxillary prosthesis has been a traditional method for rehabilitation. This not only creates an oro-nasal seal but also improves speech and swallowing. The inherent problems of maintaining hygiene and the cumbersome practice of wearing and removing the prosthesis are the key factors for dissatisfaction.

SECONDARY INTENTION, PRIMARY CLOSURE, OR LOCAL FLAP ADVANCEMENT

Small superficial soft tissue defects can be left to heal secondarily, but soft tissue or coverage with a dressing will facilitate rapid wound healing.

Primary closure seems to be a more suitable option in lower alveolus defects due to availability of mobile buccal and lingual mucosal tissue. Performing primary wound closure in the upper alveolus can be tricky, as mucosa is not very mobile and a tight closure usually results in wound dehiscence.

Local/Pedicled Flaps

Palatal Island Rotation Flap

Based on the greater palatine artery, a branch of the descending palatine artery, the palatal flap based on a single palatine artery can be used to reconstruct the defect of the posterior alveolus, the retromolar trigone, and part of the lower alveolus. The donor site can be left to heal secondarily or covered by a white head varnish dressing with minimal morbidity. The flap can be designed, leaving 5 mm of palato-gingival margins and raised subperiosteally. The arc of rotation can be increased by removing the posterolateral bone of the greater palatine foramen.

Nasolabial Flap

As described earlier, the nasolabial flap makes an ideal option in an elderly, edentulous patient for the coverage of lower or upper alveolar defects with a reach up to the midline maxillary or mandibular ridge. The flap can be done as a one- or two-staged procedure with division performed after 2 to 3 weeks.

Buccal Pad of Fat

The buccal pad of fat makes a robust option to cover the superficial, small-sized posterior maxillary, mandibular alveolus, or retromolar trigon defects. This lobulated fat has reasonably good blood supply and volume, does not atrophy much, and mucosalizes well over the period. The surgical technique involves mucosal incision while preventing injury to the Stensen's duct and divides the buccinator, allowing the buccal pad of fat to herniate through the muscle into the oral cavity. The limitation is the anterior reach of the fat, as too much advancement will result in devascularization of the fat.

Facial Artery Myomucosal Flap

Based on the anterograde or retrograde flow of the facial artery, a FAMM flap is an excellent rotational flap, providing thin and pliable tissue for alveolar ridge/FOM coverage. The limitation is the width (up to 2 cm) in order to avoid post-operative trismus or scarring at the donor site. The distal end of the flap is marked anterior to the Stensen's duct for an anterior-based flap and 1 cm posterior to the oral commissure for a posterior-based flap. A Doppler is used to locate the course of the facial artery. The incision is placed through the mucosa, submucosa, and buccinator muscle. The technique is to harvest the flap while keeping the facial artery attached to the elevated flap.

Submental Artery Flap

As discussed earlier, the submental artery flap is a new addition to the armamentarium and provides an excellent solution to medium-sized defects with reasonable bulk to reconstruct defects of the lower alveolus after mucosal resections and marginal mandibulectomy. The flap can be transferred to the oral cavity by making a tunnel either from the buccal or lingual aspect of the mandible. The flap stays under the radar due to the questionable oncological safety.

The donor site can be closed primarily. The variable venous drainage patterns and hair growth in patients not amenable to radiation therapy are the limiting factors that need to be considered while harvesting the submental artery flap.

Palatal Defects

For smaller defects involving the alveolar ridge, teeth, and surrounding mucosa, local flaps provide reasonably good coverage. Early lesions require wide local resections sparing the underlying bone but advanced disease warrants partial or subtotal/total maxillectomy creating a nasomaxillary defect requiring complex planning and reconstruction.

Mucosal Defect Only

For a mucosal defect only, a simple dressing that promotes granulation tissue formation such as white head varnish will suffice.

Soft Tissue and Bony Defect

The presence of palatal bone creates a separation between oral and nasal cavities. Loss of this support results in oro-antral communication.

Palatal Obturators

The presence or absence of dentition dictates the choice of reconstruction using local/regional flaps or a maxillofacial prosthesis. In a dentate patient, a defect resulting in maxillofacial deformity can be addressed by fabricating a palatal obturator. The benefits are short operating time, early rehabilitation, and ease of oncological follow-up. The issues related to obturators are stability, leakage of food and air in larger defects, and maintaining hygiene.

Local/Regional Flaps

Nasolabial Flap

A nasolabial flap can be used for the coverage of small anterior mucosal defects. For a larger defect, bilateral nasolabial flaps provide adequate soft tissue coverage. Unavailability of palatal bone underneath could result in wound dehiscence.

Palatal Island Flap

Rotation flaps can be used for a unilateral defect. The FAMM flap, with an average width of 1.5 × 2 cm and length of 8–9 cm can be harvested to cover the hard and soft palate defects. Sometimes, stage reconstruction is inevitable, so a pedicle can be divided in 2–3 weeks' time.

Temporalis Muscle Flap

A temporalis muscle flap is a fan-shaped flap originating along the temporal lines supplied by the anterior and posterior deep temporal arteries. The muscle has a thickness of 5 mm at the periphery and 15 m at the zygomatic arch, and up to 20 × 10 cm muscle can be used for reconstruction. The last two decades have witnessed a decrease in the use of temporalis muscle due to the emergence of free flaps as the standard of care.

The muscle can be brought into the oral cavity utilizing two approaches:

- Under the zygomatic arch that sometimes needs osteotomy
- Over the zygomatic arch but with decreased reach

The drawback of temporalis muscle is temporal hollowing, which can be camouflaged by hair growth.

CLINICAL CASES

Case 4.1

A middle-aged male had been diagnosed with SCC involving the left maxillary tuberosity area with extension into retromolar trigone. Wide local resection was performed. The palatal flap based on the ipsilateral greater palatine was raised to cover the defect while the donor site wound was packed with white head varnish for 2 weeks (Figures 4.1–4.4).

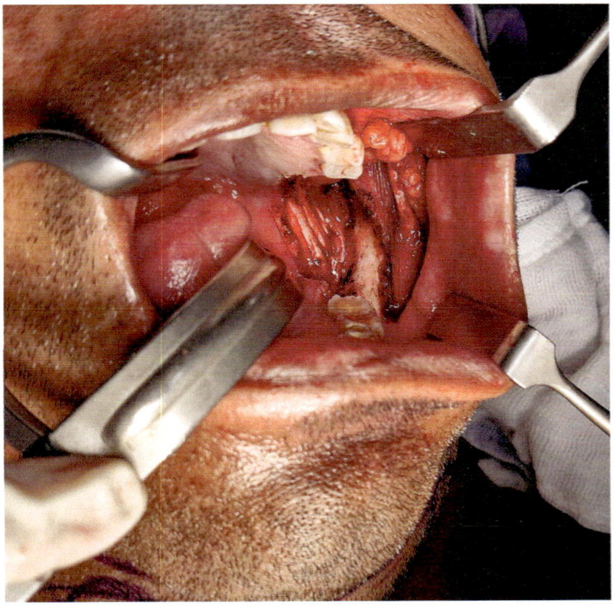

FIGURE 4.1 Tuberosity/RMT defect with exposed anterior defect following excision.

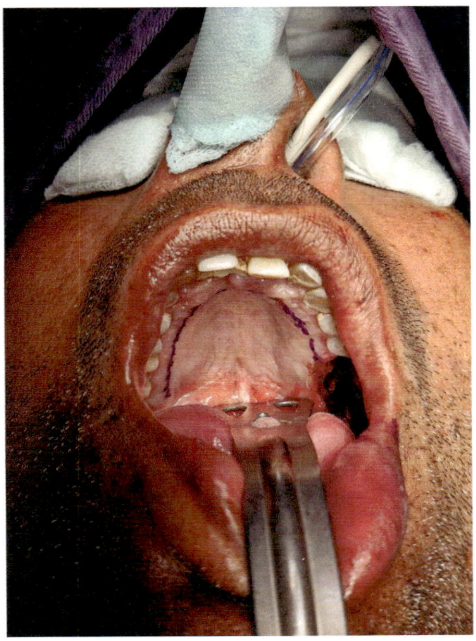

FIGURE 4.2 Markings for a palatal flap based on the left greater palatine artery and sparing 5 mm palatal gingiva.

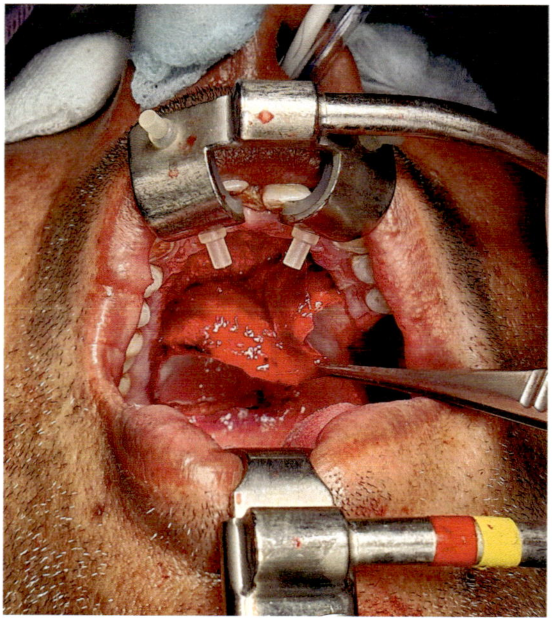

FIGURE 4.3 Subperiosteal elevation. The right greater palatine and sphenopalatine artery are ligated.

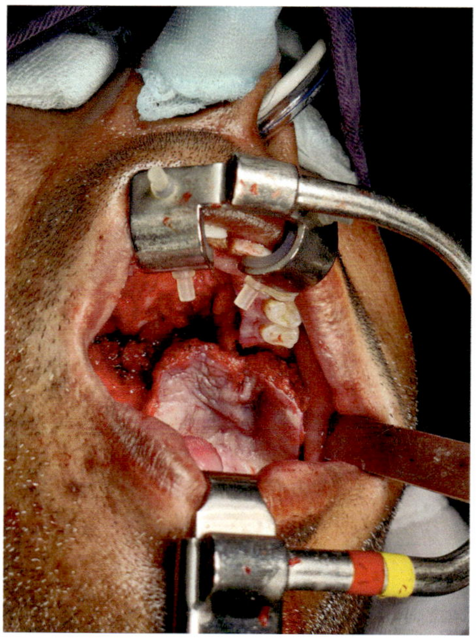

FIGURE 4.4 Palatal flap is rotated to cover the defect.

Case 4.2

A 63-year-old male, with a known case of SCC lower labial sulcus with extension to alveolar mucosa but sparing the bone, was subjected to wide local resection and a marginal mandibulectomy. The defect was reconstructed using bilateral nasolabial flaps in a staged procedure. Division of the flap was performed after 2 weeks (Figures 4.5–4.10).

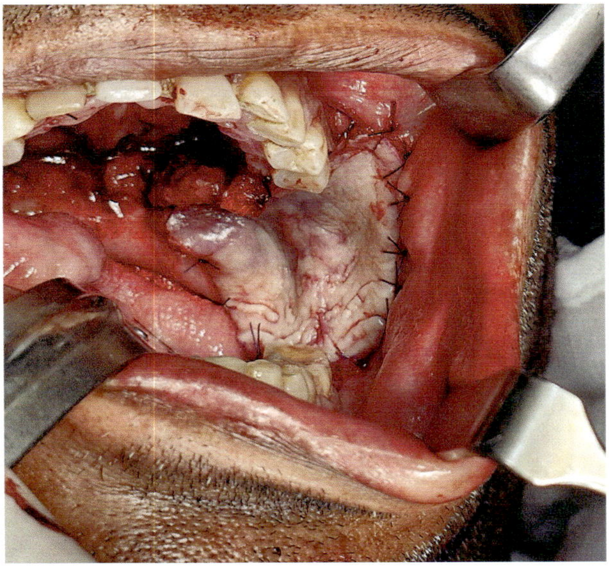

FIGURE 4.5 Flap sutured; donor site covered with white head varnish.

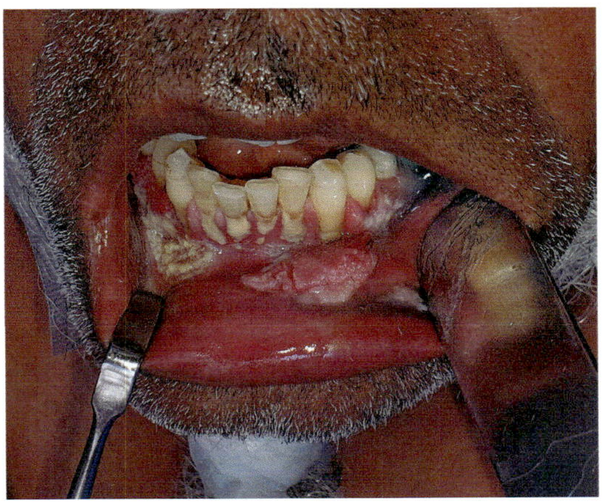

FIGURE 4.6 Anterior labial sulcus tumor involving mucosa but no bony involvement.

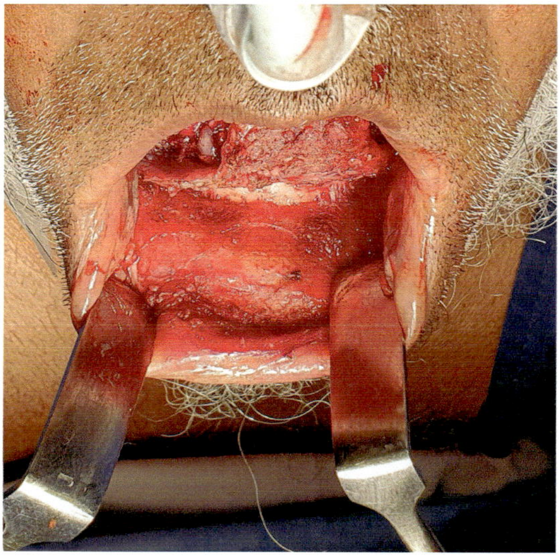

FIGURE 4.7 Defect involving labial, alveolar, and lingual mucosa.

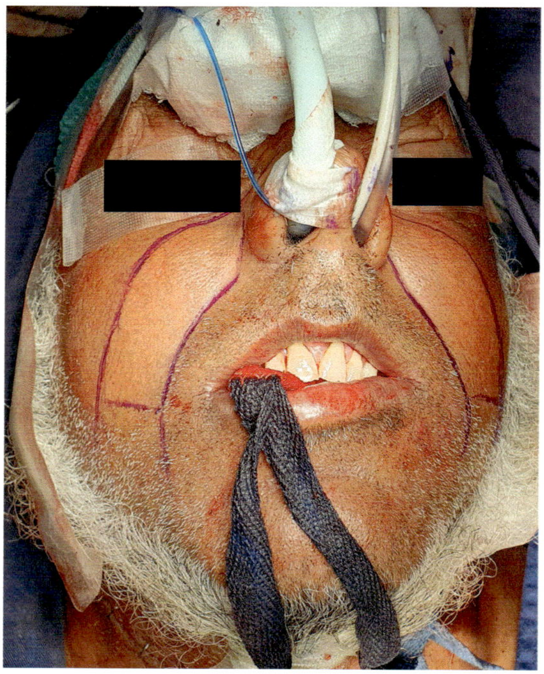

FIGURE 4.8 Design of bilateral nasolabial flaps in accordance with the mesiodistal and AP dimension of the defect.

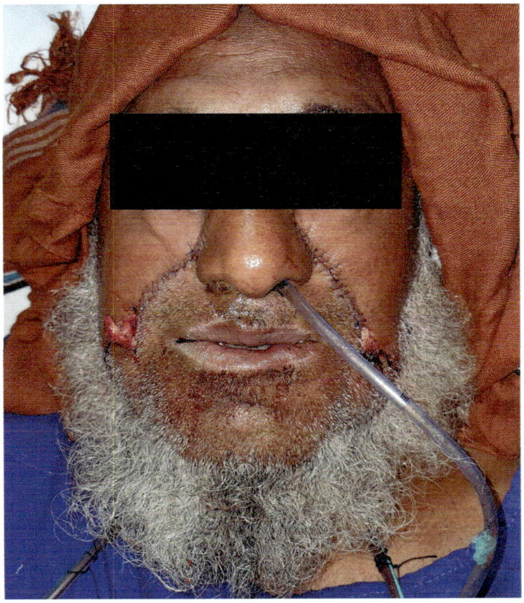

FIGURE 4.9 Primary closure at the donor site. Paraffin gauze placed at the inferior end until flap division in 2 weeks.

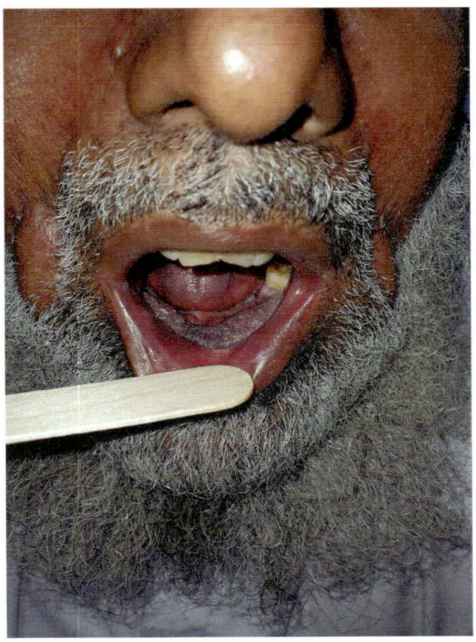

FIGURE 4.10 Wound healing 5 weeks after flap division.

Case 4.3

A 50 year old had post-operative radiotherapy for mandibular SCC and developed exposed plate and skin breakdown. The skin and plate were removed, and a left deltopectoral flap was used for coverage (Figures 4.11–4.15).

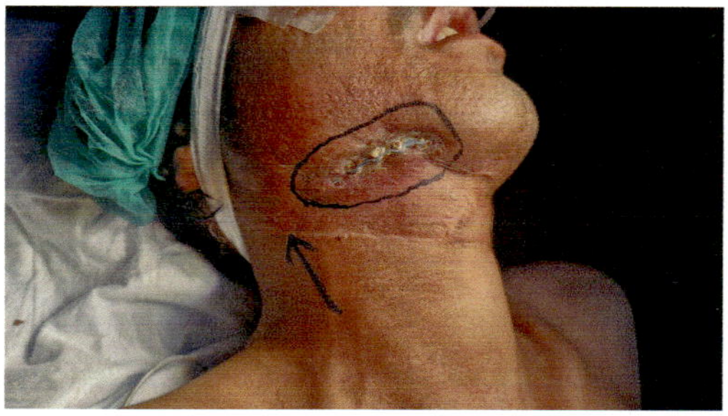

FIGURE 4.11 Exposed plate and tissue breakdown. Post-radiotherpy.

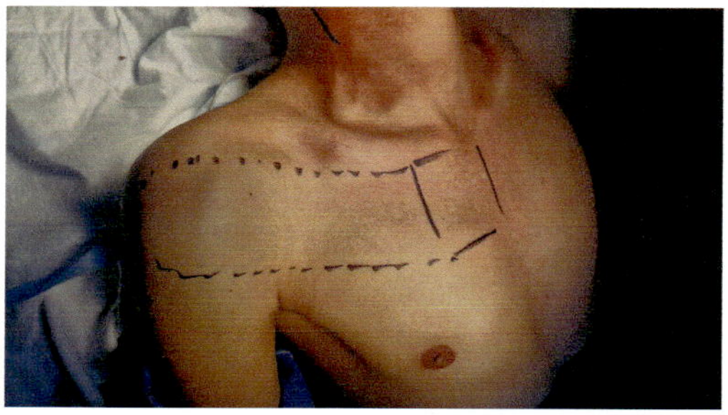

FIGURE 4.12 Skin markings for deltopectoral flap.

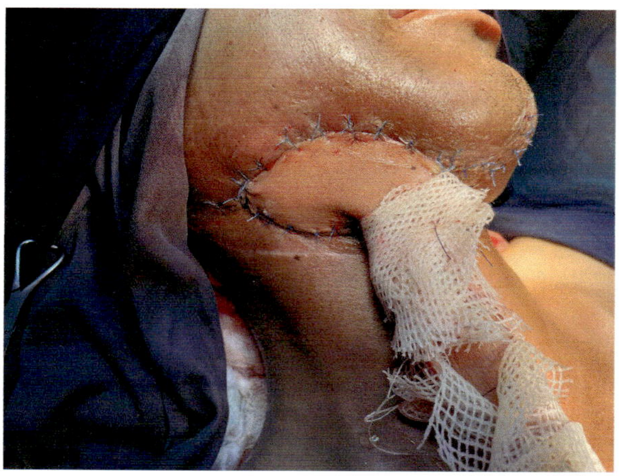

FIGURE 4.13 Flap inset and Jelonet dressing to exposed areas.

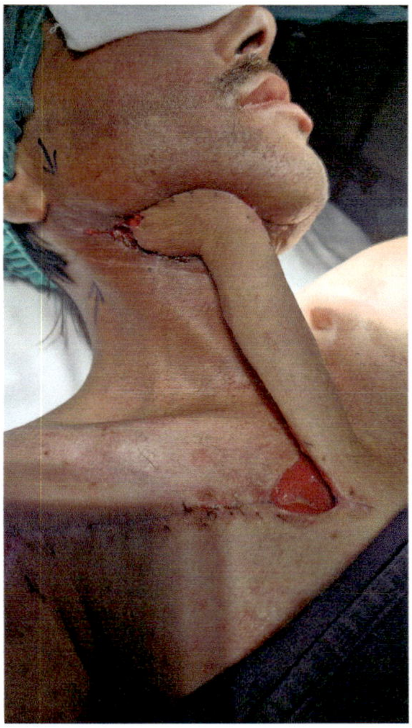

FIGURE 4.14 Stage 2 of the disconnecting flap 4 weeks post-operative.

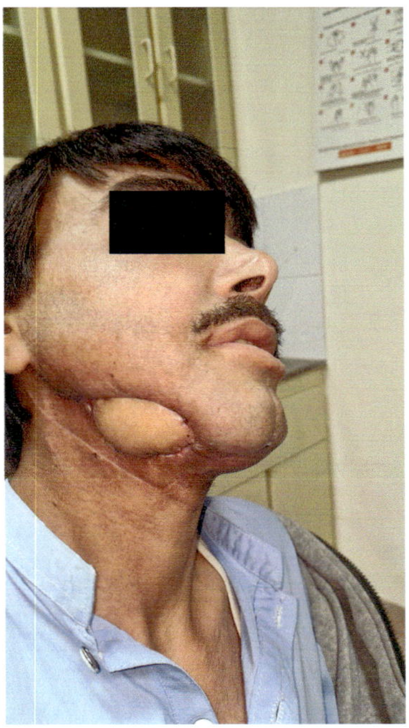

FIGURE 4.15 Well-healed wound 8 weeks post-operative.

Case 4.4

A 45-year-old male with histopathologically proven stage IV SCC of the left mandible and alveolar mucosa, extending to the condylar neck, treated with a lip split, segmental mandibulectomy, and SND, followed by reconstruction with a pectoralis major flap with no plate (Figures 4.16–4.19).

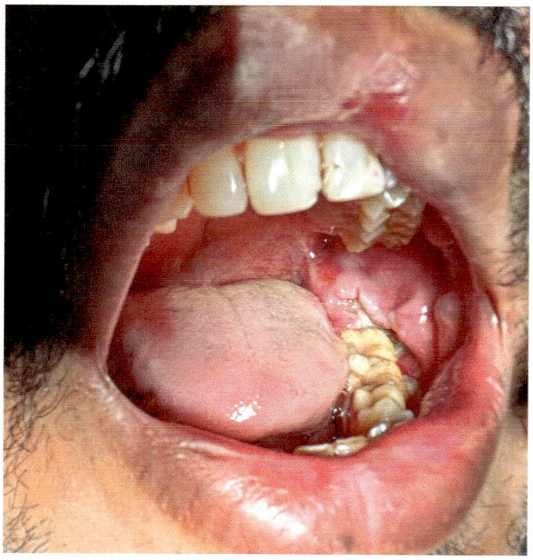

FIGURE 4.16 Primary disease on the left mandible and RMT.

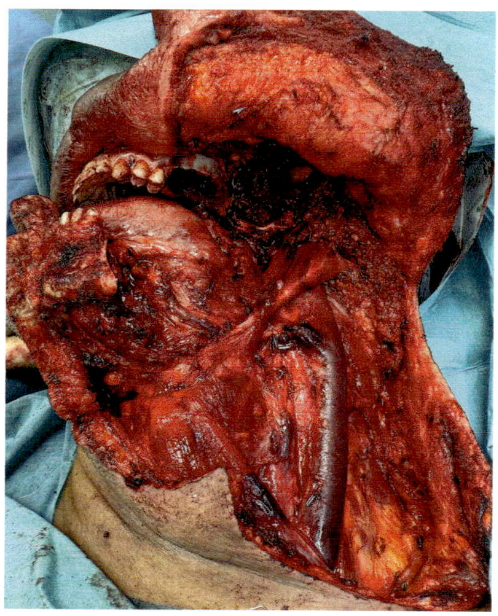

FIGURE 4.17 Wide local excision with a lip split, hemi-mandibulectomy, and removal of condylar head.

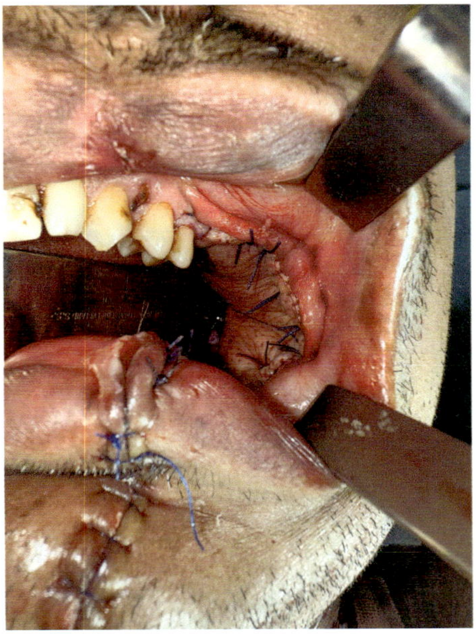

FIGURE 4.18 Pectoralis major flap inset. No plate was used.

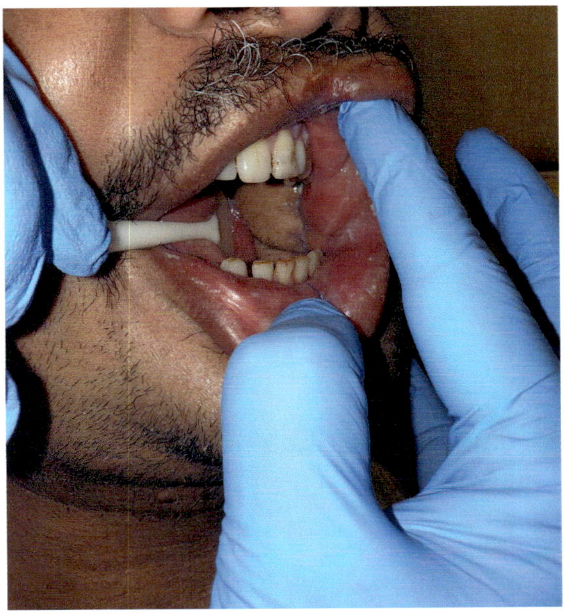

FIGURE 4.19 Six weeks post-operative, with good mouth opening and very little swing.

Case 4.5

A 60-year-old female with T4 SCC right maxilla, betel nut chewer underwent partial maxillectomy and reconstruction with an inferior-based nasolabial flap (Figures 4.20–4.23).

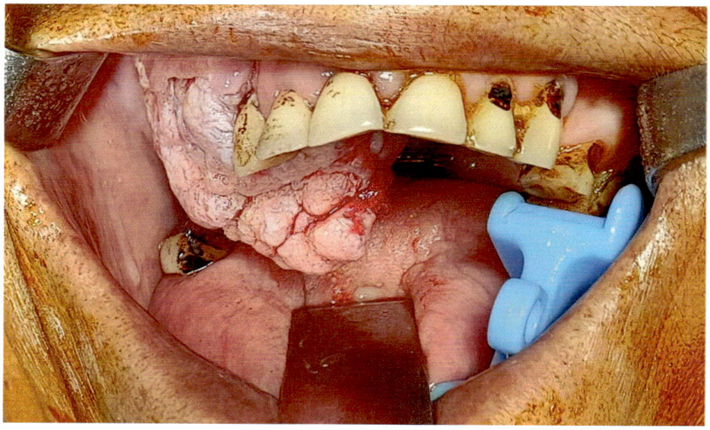

FIGURE 4.20 T4 SCC right maxilla.

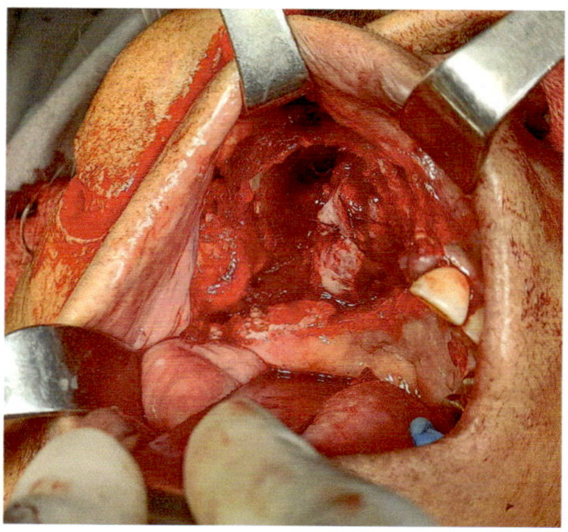

FIGURE 4.21 Partial maxillectomy.

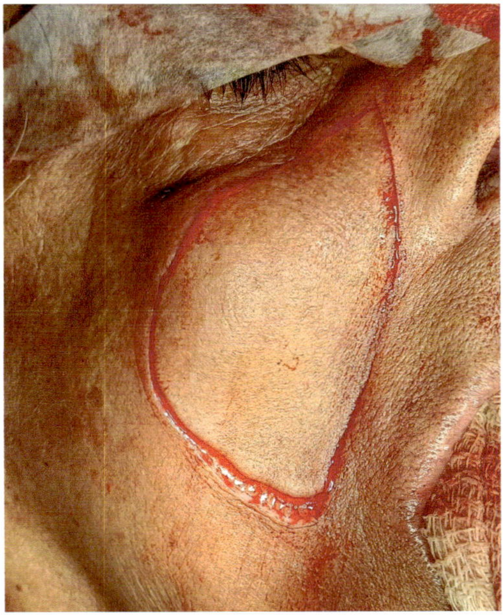

FIGURE 4.22 Inferiorly based nasolabial flap.

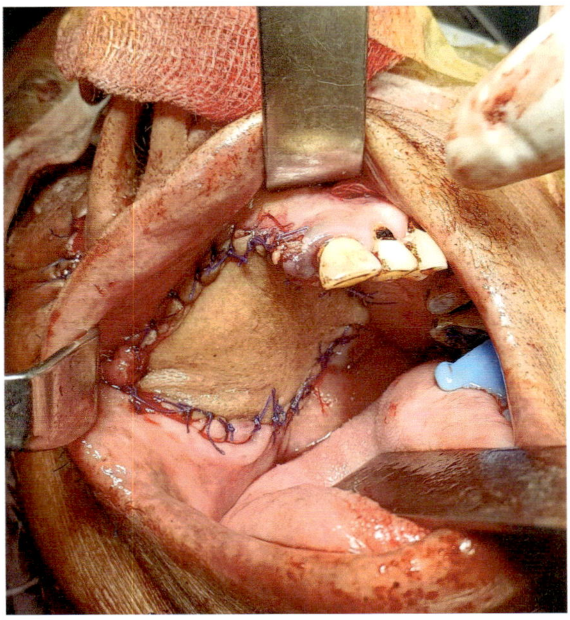

FIGURE 4.23 Flap inset.

Case 4.6

A 64-year-old male had been diagnosed with SCC involving the anterior maxilla. The patient underwent an anterior maxillectomy followed by reconstruction using bilateral nasolabial flaps as a single-stage procedure. Post-operative lip support and oro-nasal seal were the achieved objectives (Figures 4.24–4.27).

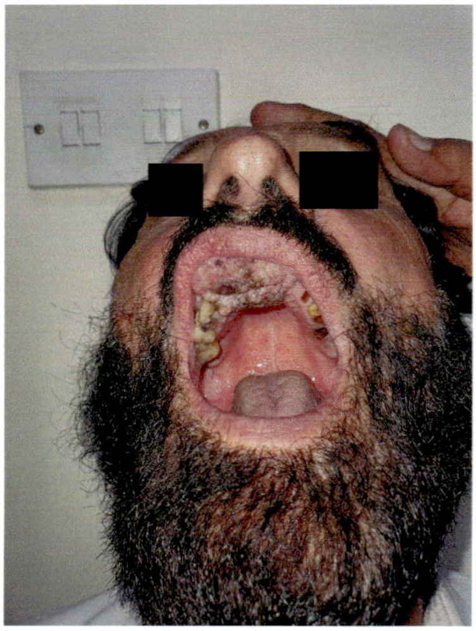

FIGURE 4.24 SCC anterior alveolus involving labial sulcus and anterior palatal mucosa.

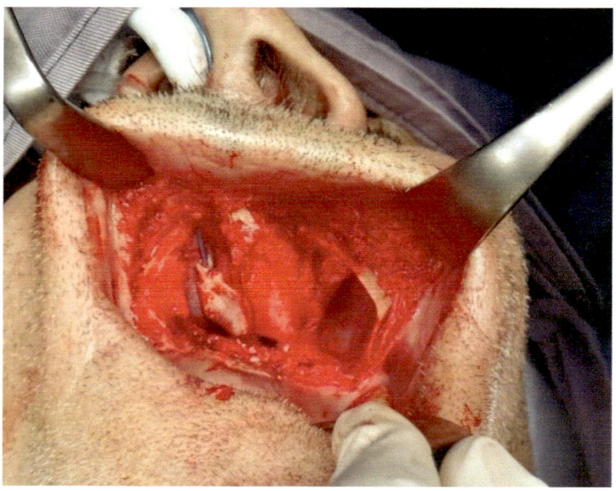

FIGURE 4.25 Post-maxillectomy defect showing nasal septum and left maxillary sinus.

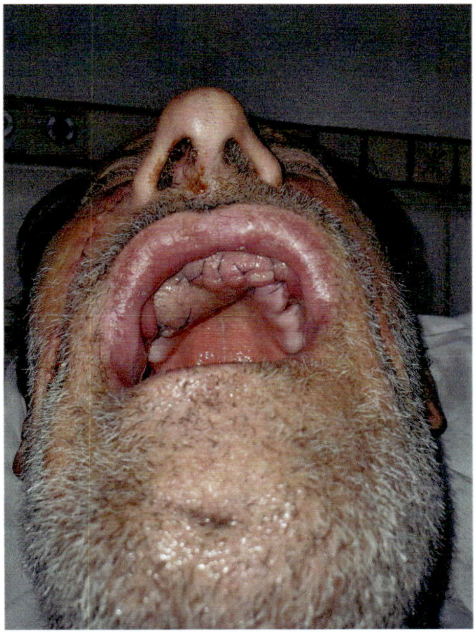

FIGURE 4.26 Bilateral nasolabial flaps with their medial borders sutured in the midline.

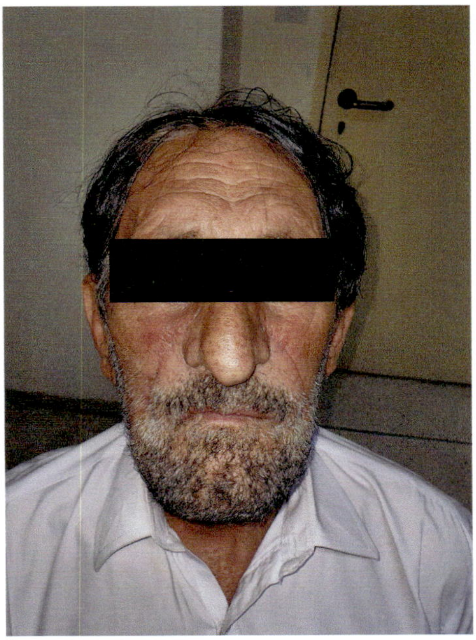

FIGURE 4.27 Twelve months post-operative: Good mouth opening and lip support.

Case 4.7

An 85 year old with T1 maxillary carcinoma treated with excision and buccal fat pad, good mouth opening, and no disease recurrence 2 years post-operative (Figures 4.28–4.30).

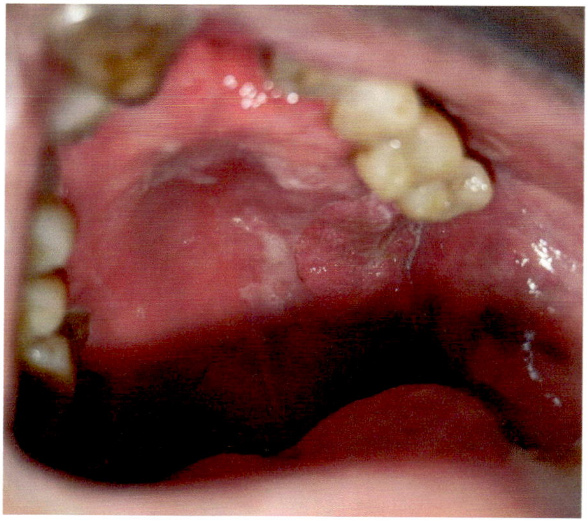

FIGURE 4.28 T1 SCC left maxilla.

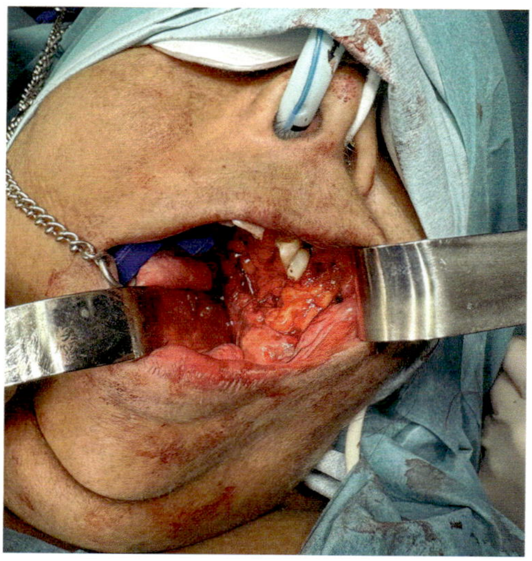

FIGURE 4.29 Buccal fat pad.

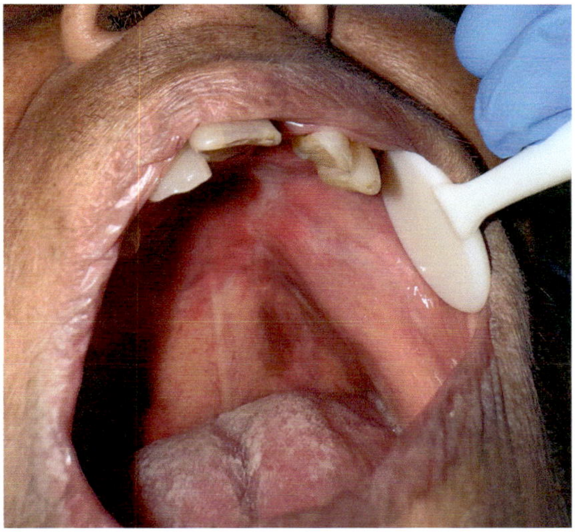

FIGURE 4.30 One-year post-operative.

Case 4.8

A 45-year-old male was diagnosed with SCC in the left lower alveolus, extending to involve the left labial sulcus/buccal mucosa and facial skin. The patient underwent wide local resection, segmental mandibulectomy, and neck dissection. The defect required both internal and external lining. A left-sided submental flap was used to reconstruct the defect (Figures 4.31–4.35).

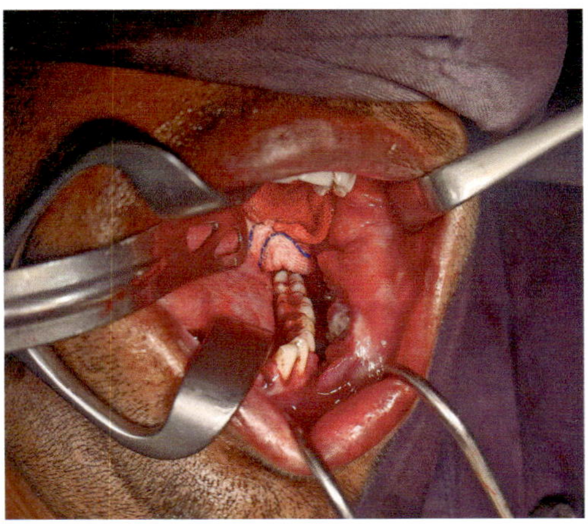

FIGURE 4.31 SCC left mandible and alveolus.

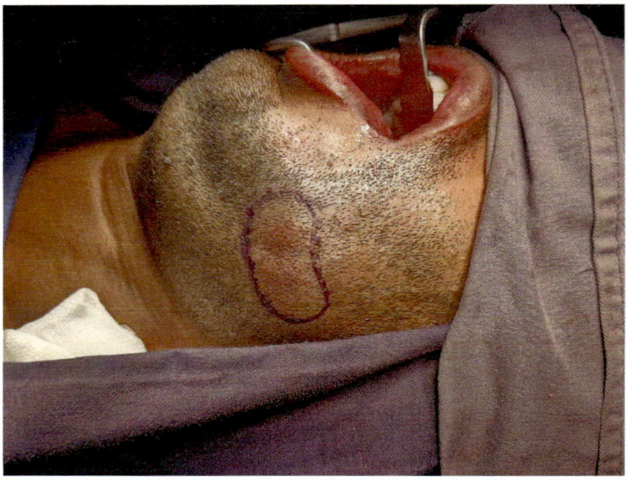

FIGURE 4.32 Skin tethering noted.

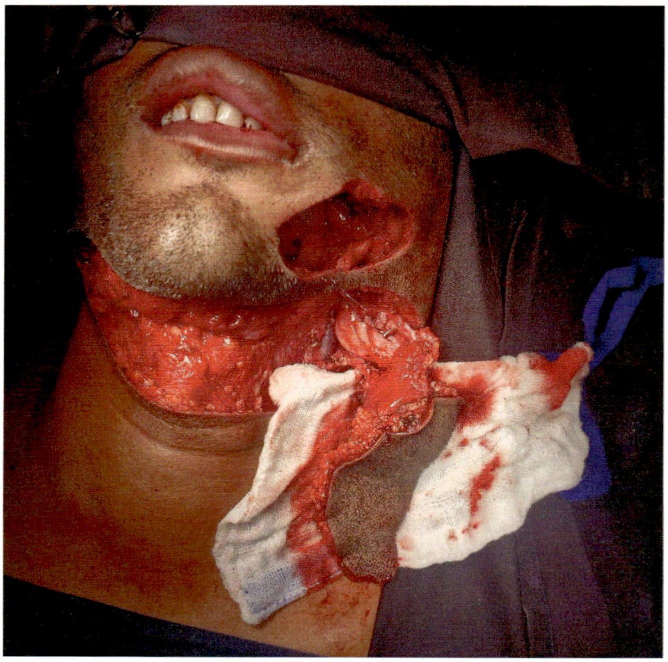

FIGURE 4.33 Segmental mandibulectomy, with skin and left submental flap raised.

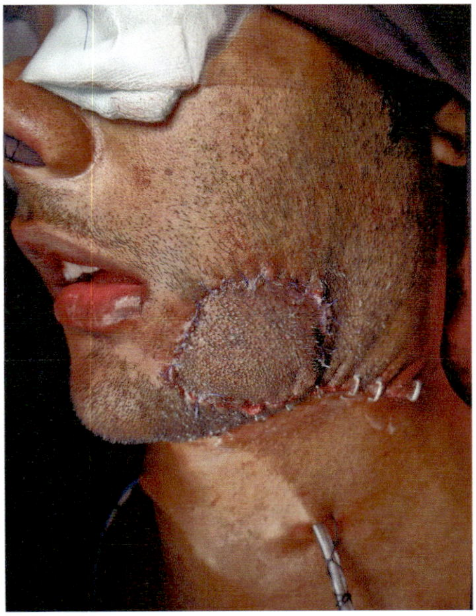

FIGURE 4.34 Submental flap inset to cover oral and skin lining.

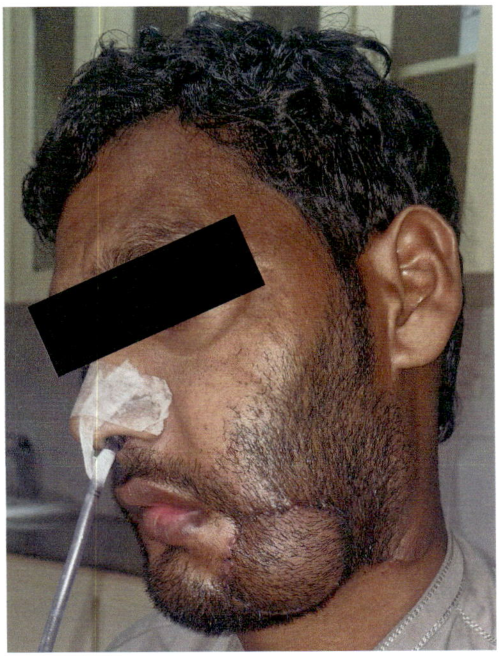

FIGURE 4.35 Two weeks post-operative.

Case 4.9

A 57-year-old male developed carcinoma in the left lower anterior alveolus. An infrahyoid flap with a 7 × 3 cm skin island (allowing primary closure of the donor site) was planned. Left segmental mandibulectomy and neck dissection were performed, while the flap was elevated based on the superior thyroid vessels (Figures 4.36–4.39).

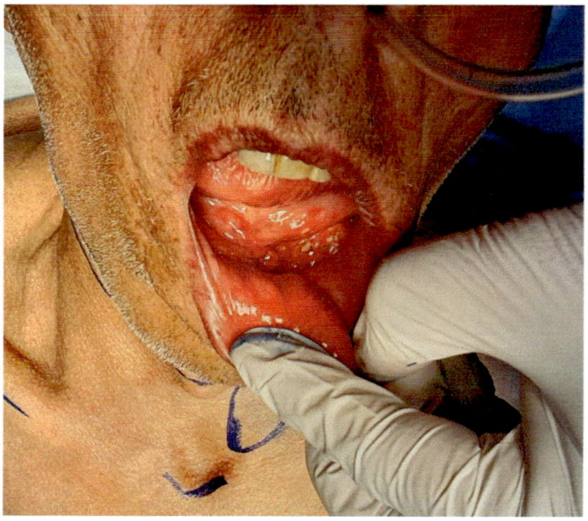

FIGURE 4.36 Left lower alveolus tumor in an edentulous lower ridge.

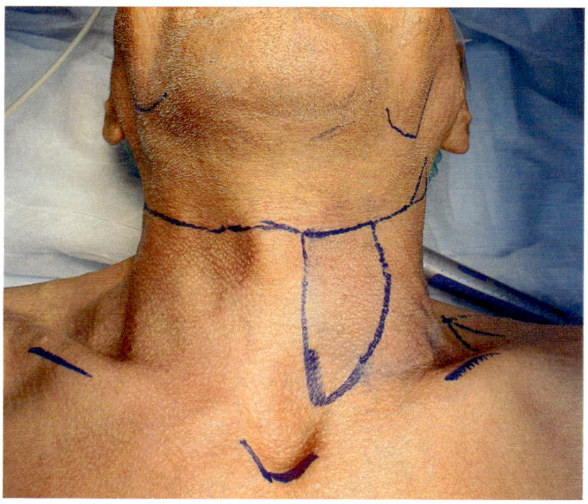

FIGURE 4.37 Design of infrahyoid muscle flap with a 7 × 3 cm skin component for primary donor site closure.

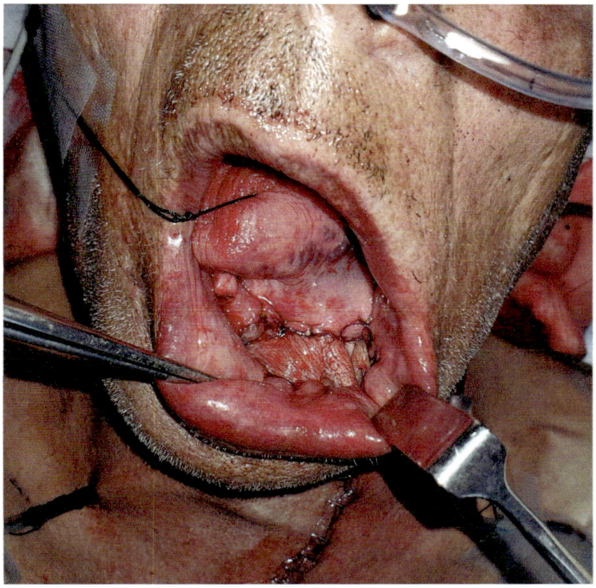

FIGURE 4.38 Flap sutured to the labial and lingual mucosa post-segmental mandibulectomy.

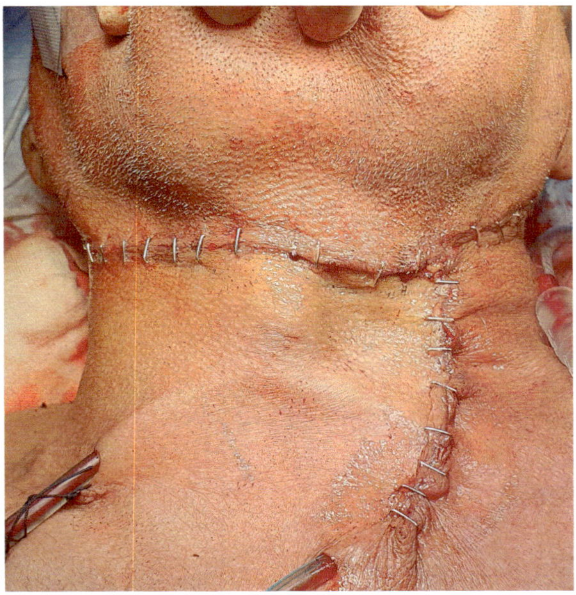

FIGURE 4.39 Closure of the donor site.

Case 4.10

A 60 year old with SCC of the left palate and alveolus underwent a maxillectomy with partial closure with buccal fat pad and white head varnish pack (Figures 4.40–4.42).

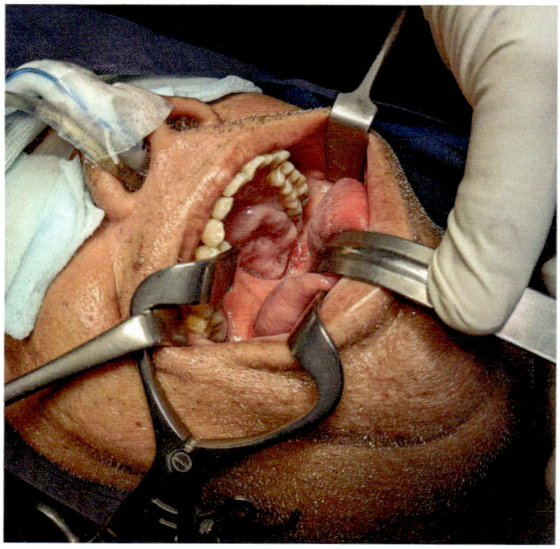

FIGURE 4.40 SCC left maxilla and palate.

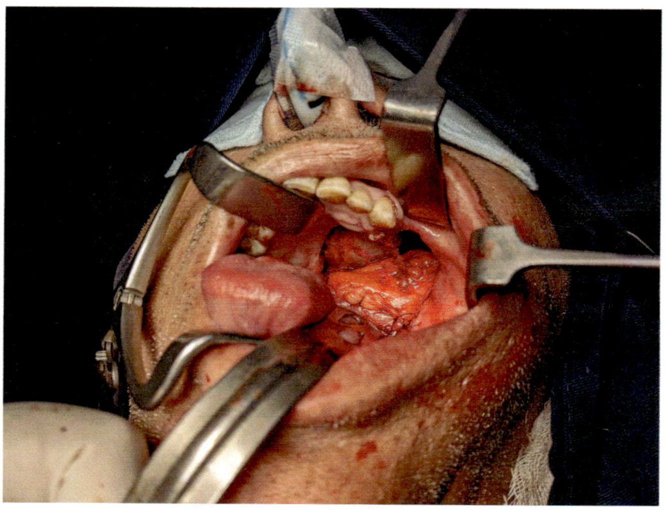

FIGURE 4.41 Resection and buccal fat pad raised.

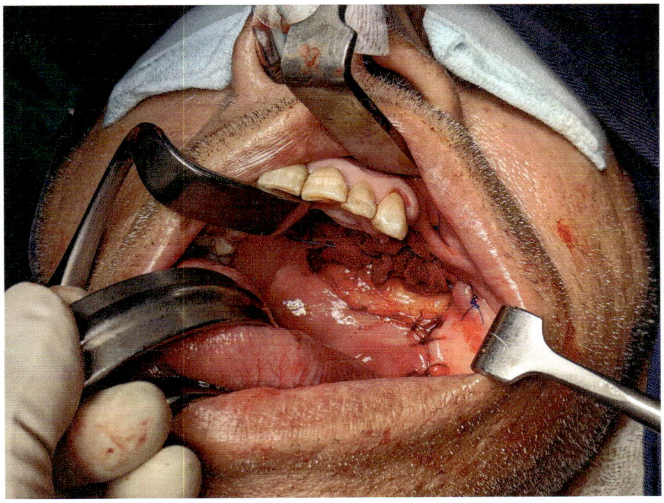

FIGURE 4.42 Post-operative, using a buccal fat pad and white head varnish pack.

Case 4.11

A 70 year old with SCC of the anterior maxilla and alveolus underwent partial maxillectomy and reconstruction with bilateral nasolabial flaps (Figures 4.43–4.47).

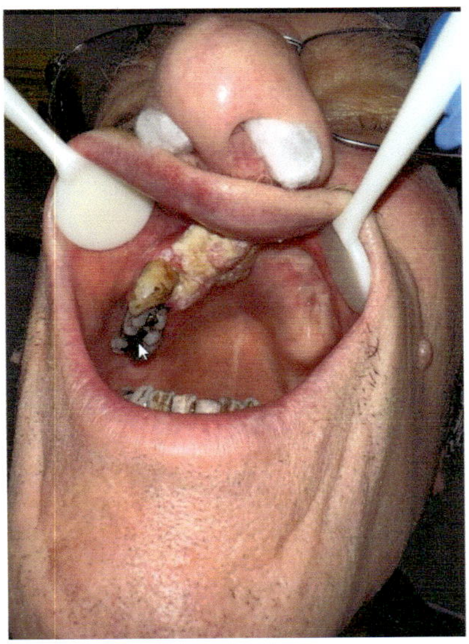

FIGURE 4.43 SCC anterior maxilla.

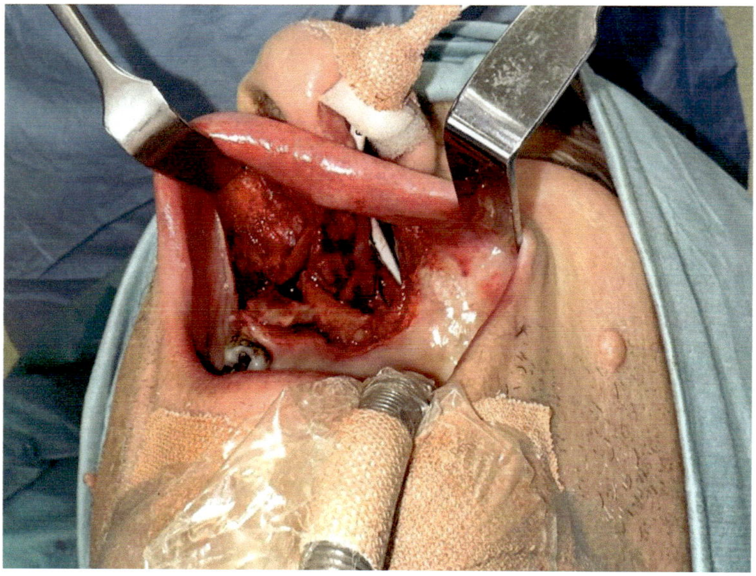

FIGURE 4.44 Partia aterior maxillectomy.

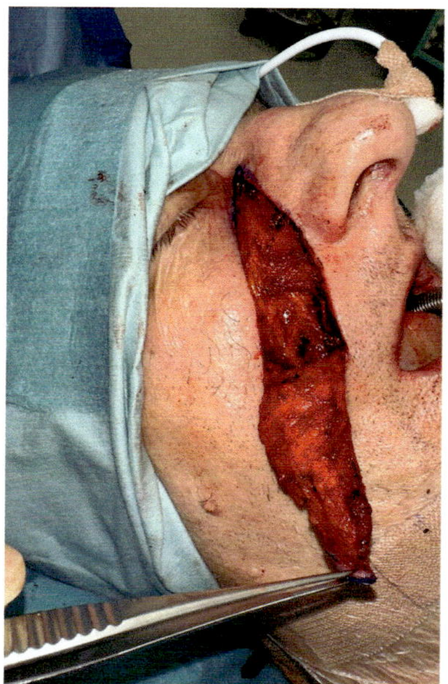

FIGURE 4.45 Nasolabial flap raised.

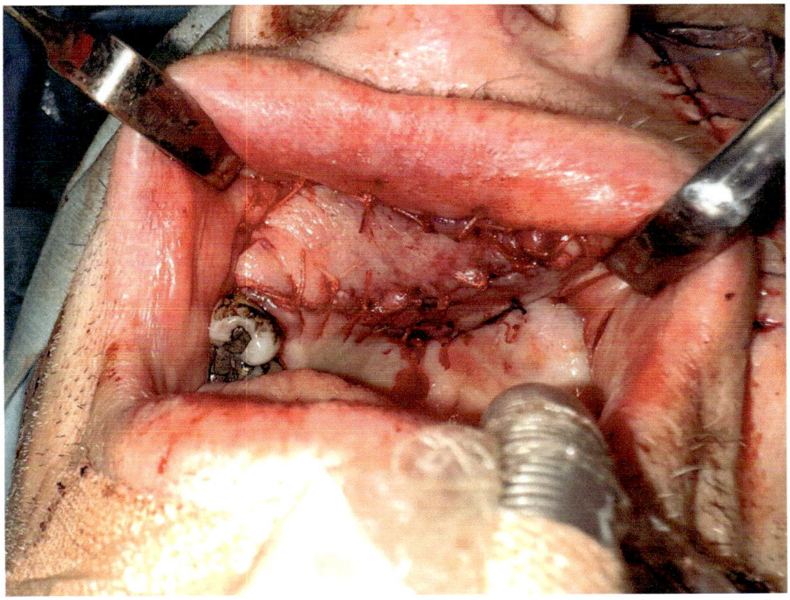

FIGURE 4.46 Nasolbail flap inset.

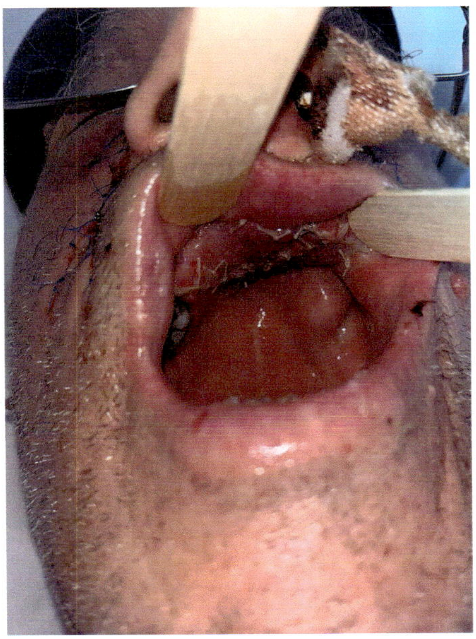

FIGURE 4.47 Two weeks post-operative.

Case 4.12

A 65 year old underwent partial maxillectomy and reconstruction with a nasolabial flap (Figures 4.48 and 4.49).

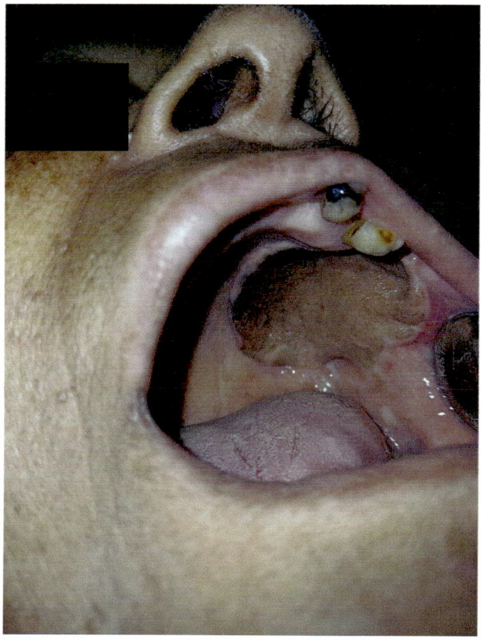

FIGURE 4.48 Healed nasolabial reconstruction for partial maxillectomy.

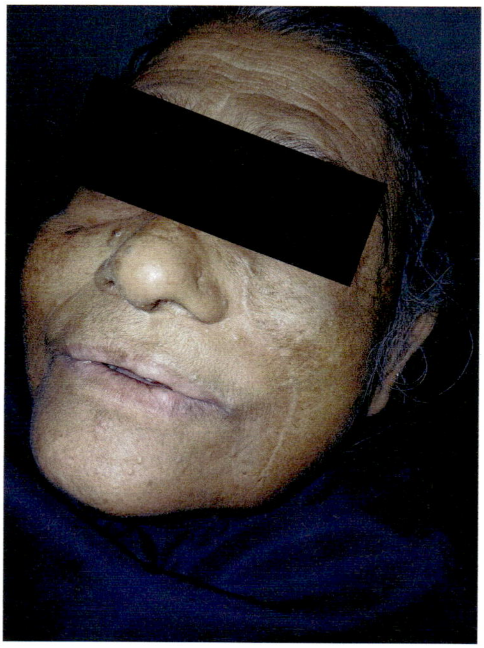

FIGURE 4.49 External scar.

Case 4.13

A 70 year old had a segmental mandibulectomy and partial glossectomy. Reconstruction with the pectoralis major flap (Figures 4.50–4.53).

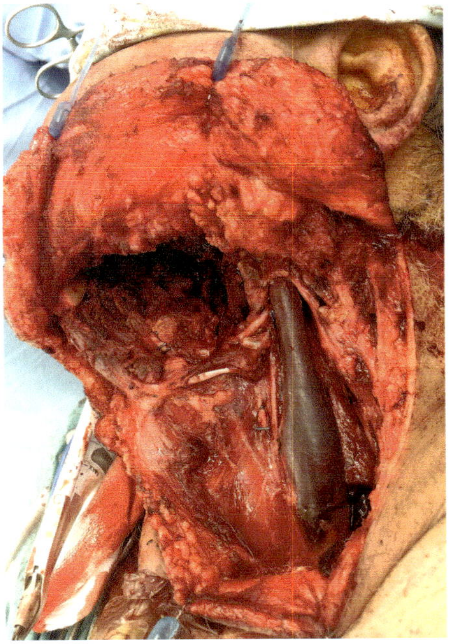

FIGURE 4.50 Left segmental mandibulectomy and partial glossectomy.

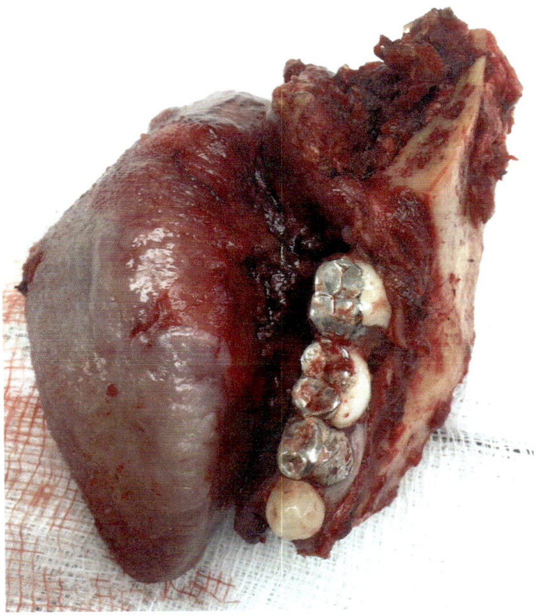

FIGURE 4.51 Specimen.

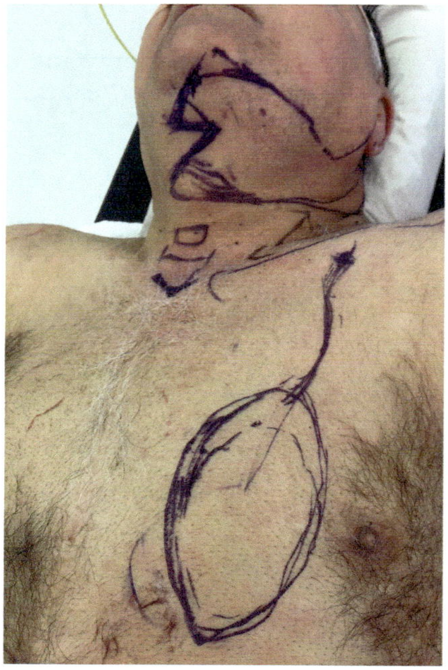

FIGURE 4.52 Marking of the pectoralis major flap.

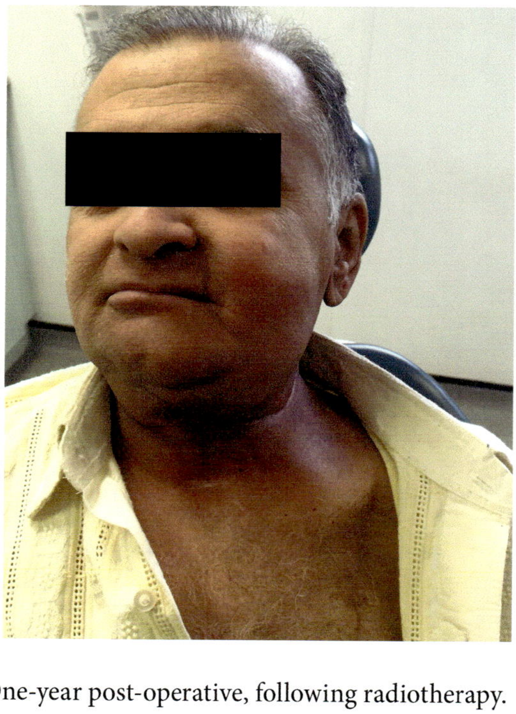

FIGURE 4.53 One-year post-operative, following radiotherapy.

Case 4.14

An elderly patient with a small T1, right maxilla, underwent a right partial maxillectomy and reconstruction with a buccal fat pad (Figures 4.54–4.56).

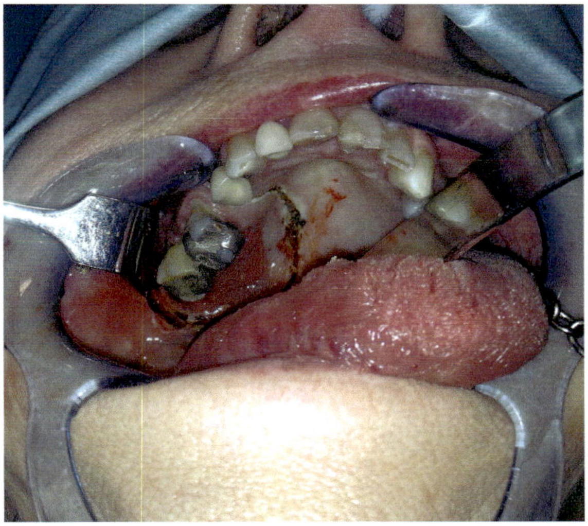

FIGURE 4.54 Partial maxillectomy of SCC for a small T1.

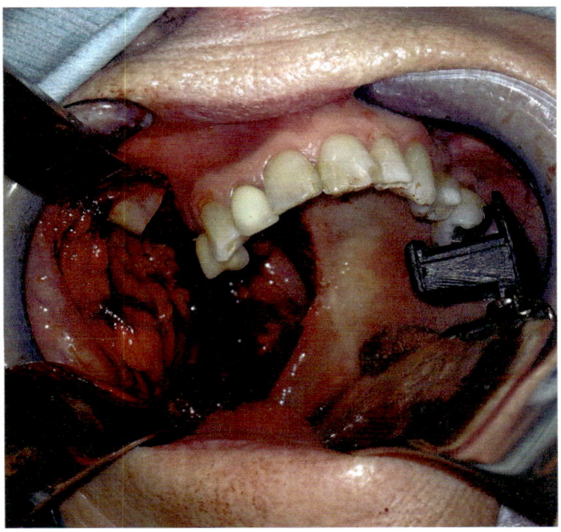

FIGURE 4.55 Mobilization of the buccal fat pad.

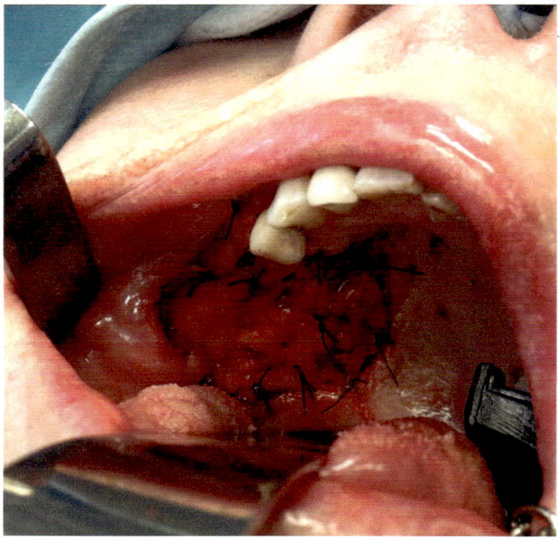

FIGURE 4.56 Full closure of defect using a buccal fat pad.

DISCUSSION

Resection of the upper alveolus or palate often results in defects that present significant challenges, such as oro-nasal or oro-antral communication; loss of support for the lip, cheek, or periorbita; and difficulties with dysphagia and speech. The primary reconstructive goals include closing the sinus defect, restoring the separation between the oral and nasal or oral and sinus cavities, and reestablishing facial contours. Conventional maxillary prostheses are commonly used to obturate the defect and achieve an oro-nasal or oro-antral seal, with the added benefit of including dentition to enhance both aesthetics and chewing function. However, these prostheses require regular cleaning for hygiene and periodic adjustments to address leakage and surface irregularities.

The choice of flap for reconstruction depends on factors, such as the extent of the defect, patient-specific considerations, and the surgeon's expertise. Local flaps are typically used for small defects due to their simplicity and minimal morbidity, while larger or more complex defects often necessitate regional flaps.

For unilateral soft tissue defects of the upper alveolus that extend to the midline, the ipsilateral nasolabial flap provides the necessary reach and bulk. For mucosal defects crossing the midline, bilateral nasolabial flaps can be employed. Major defects resulting from the loss of alveolus or palatal bone may be reconstructed using the temporalis flap, which offers adequate bulk and coverage. The palatal flap is also a reliable option for smaller palatal defects, though it is limited by its arc of rotation and the need for antiseptic dressing to cover the palate.

For lower alveolus mucosal defects, nasolabial flaps can be utilized to cover the underlying bone, with the donor site defect typically closed by de-epithelializing the proximal third of the skin at the flap base. This technique also eliminates the need for flap division 2 to 3 weeks later. The nasolabial flap offers sufficient bulk to cover defects from marginal mandibulectomy.

The FAMM flap is effective for covering mucosal defects in the lower alveolus, while the buccal pad of fat is a suitable alternative for small posterior lower alveolus or retromolar trigone defects, provided excessive stretch is avoided to prevent fat atrophy.

For larger defects involving the lower alveolar bone requiring segmental mandibulectomy, a bulky flap is necessary to restore facial form and prevent oro-cervical communication. The pectoralis major flap provides the required bulk, and other potential options include submental and supraclavicular flaps. The presence of positive level 1 nodes with clinical extra-nodal extension (ENE) or involvement of the facial artery contraindicates the use of a submental flap. However, large but mobile level 1 nodes without clinical ENE can be removed without compromising the vascularity of the submental flap. In cases of clinically positive nodes (cN+), the use of the submental flap remains a decision for the primary surgeon.

When facial skin involvement accompanies lower alveolar defects and free flap reconstruction is not viable due to resource limitations, expertise, or medical conditions, a combination of local and regional flaps can be considered. Small focal defects of the overlying facial skin may not require a flap and can be closed primarily. Medium-sized defects can be reconstructed with bi-paddled pectoralis major or submental flaps. In some cases, two local flaps can be used to provide both internal and external coverage.

CHAPTER 5

Floor of the Mouth

KEY POINTS

- **Anatomical Complexity and Surgical Challenges**: The floor of the mouth (FOM) is a complex, anatomically confined space surrounded by critical structures, making surgical resection challenging. Achieving clear margins is often complicated by early tumor invasion into adjacent structures, such as the mandible and deep tongue muscles.
- **Reconstructive Options and Functional Preservation**: Reconstruction is essential for maintaining oral function after FOM tumor resection. For smaller defects, local flaps like the nasolabial or FAMM flap may suffice to restore both function and aesthetics.
- **Neck Dissection and Radiotherapy Controversies**: Due to the high risk of regional metastasis, routine neck dissection is commonly recommended. There is ongoing debate over whether surgery or radiotherapy offers better outcomes for neck management, with considerations around morbidity and recurrence rates.
- **Post-Operative Function and Quality of Life**: FOM tumors significantly impact speech and swallowing, and the choice of reconstructive technique affects post-operative quality of life. Rehabilitation, including physiotherapy, speech therapy, and dietary modifications, is crucial for functional recovery.

The FOM is a mucosal-lined space overlying the mylohyoid and hyoglossus muscles, with the sublingual gland lying in the lateral FOM and papillae of submandibular gland opening in the anteromedial FOM. The region is divided into right and left halves by the lingual frenulum. The lymphatic

DOI: 10.1201/9781032714585-5

drainage is to the submental, perifacial (pre- and post-vascular), sub-digastric, and jugulodigastric nodes with increased risk of bilateral drainage.

The intact FOM is critical for normal functioning of the oral tongue. The absence of intact mucosa results in compromised tongue mobility and oro-cervical communication in the case of deeper resections when combined with neck dissections.

An important aspect of FOM reconstruction is the timing. The delay usually allows surgical fibrosis to set in, causing wound contracture. A mobile tissue prevents tethering of the tongue to the fixed gingiva.

More than 90% of FOM cancers are SCC with sublingual gland malignancies, minor salivary gland tumors, sarcomas, and melanomas in the list of differentials.

The anatomical location of the FOM makes it prone to pooling of carcinogens and increased contact time to noxious substances. Whether this exposure and contact to carcinogen time translates into increased risk has yet to be established.

The treatment of a FOM tumor depends upon:

- Size
- Stage
- Involvement of adjacent anatomical structures
    - Mucosa
    - Muscle
    - Bone
- Mandible/tongue/sublingual/submandibular gland

RECONSTRUCTIVE GOALS

- Thin, pliable tissue to allow mobility of the tongue.
- Creating a partition to prevent oro-cervical communication.

HEALING BY SECONDARY INTENTION/ANTISEPTIC DRESSING/SKIN GRAFT

The superficial leukoplakic, ulcerative lesions involving FOM mucosa only and sparing underlying muscle can be managed by wide local excision and can be left to heal secondarily. In order to prevent post-surgical fibrosis and tethering of the tongue, workable solutions include white head varnish dressing (which promotes granulation tissue) or a split-thickness skin graft with bolster dressing.

Nasolabial Flap

The nasolabial flap is a reliable option for elderly patients with edentulous status. It can be done as a single or staged procedure. For smaller defects, an ipsilateral flap provides adequate tissue, while large anteroposterior or mediolateral defects can be managed by bilateral nasolabial flaps.

Facial Artery Myomucosal Flap

With an inherent limitation of width, the facial artery myomucosal flap is an excellent option because of its thin, pliable nature for reconstruction of FOM defects. The anterior-based flap provides better reach and arc of rotation for defects extending to the contralateral FOM.

Submental Flap

The fasciocutaneous submental flap is also considered to be an option in the list of locoregional flaps for oral cavity defects. The FIN SCC has the highest propensity to metastasize to the submental (level 1A) lymph nodes. The use of a submental flap has the inherent risk of jeopardizing the oncological safety of the procedure. Additionally, the thickness of the flap may not be ideal in an area which needs relatively thin and pliable tissue.

Pectoralis Major Flap

The FOM defects involving extensive resections such as underlying musculature (mylohyoid, genioglossus, hyoglossus, digastric) along with the anterior mandible can be managed by utilizing a pectoralis major musculocutaneous flap along with a reconstruction plate to stabilize the mandible. The only drawback is that the majority of these patients, when subjected to radiation therapy, were found to have exposure of the underlying plate.

CLINICAL CASES

Case 5.1

A 61-year-old female with a verrucous SCC left FOM (T2N0) underwent wide local excision, neck dissection, and reconstruction with a facial artery musculo-mucosal flap. A small rim of the mandible was taken. The patient was edentulous. She made an excellent recovery with good mouth opening (Figures 5.1–5.5).

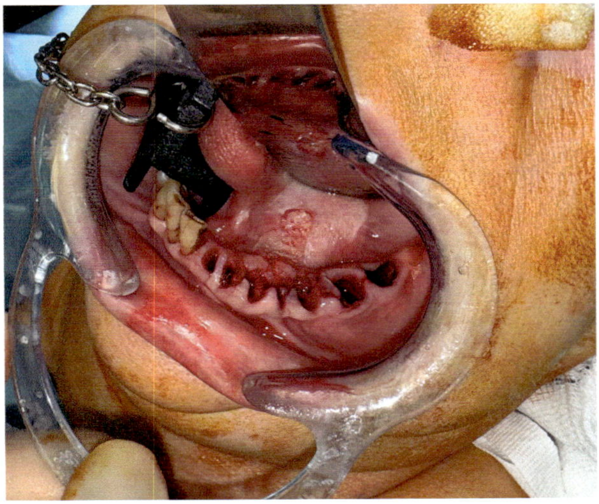

FIGURE 5.1 Tumor visualized after teeth extraction.

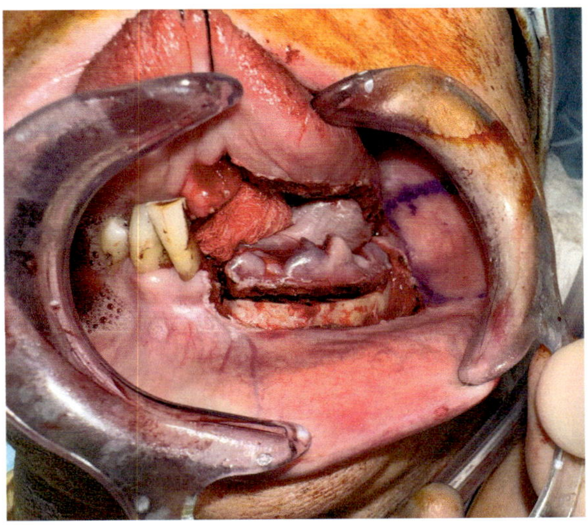

FIGURE 5.2 Mandibular ridge taken as part of the surgical margin.

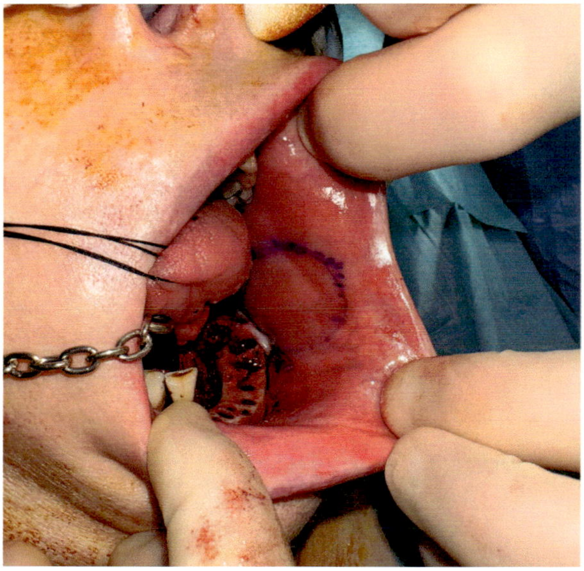

FIGURE 5.3 Design of the FAMM flap.

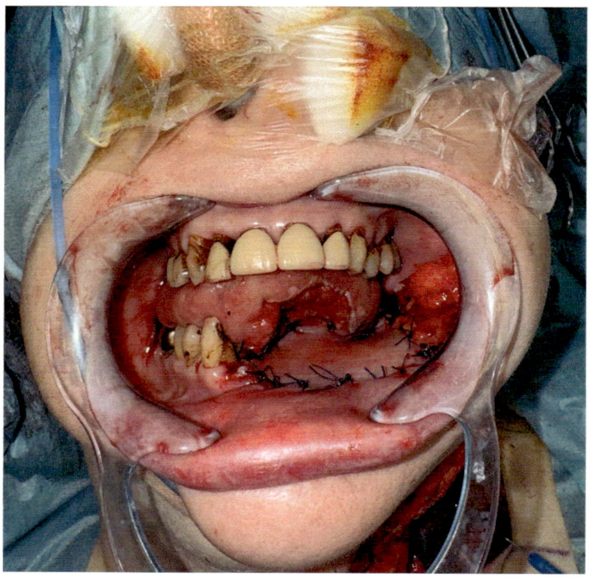

FIGURE 5.4 Immediately post-operative. Donor site closed with a buccal fat pad.

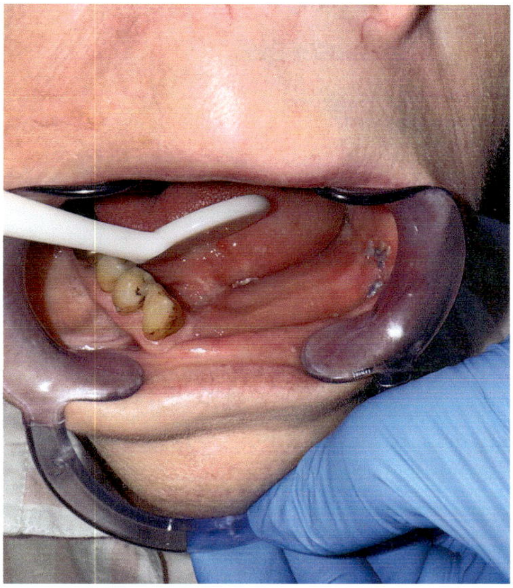

FIGURE 5.5 Three months post-operative.

Case 5.2

A 67-year-old male with a history of excessive alcohol consumption presented with anterior midline FOM SCC. He underwent a wide local excision, bilateral neck dissection, and reconstruction with a bilateral nasolabial flap (Figures 5.6–5.9).

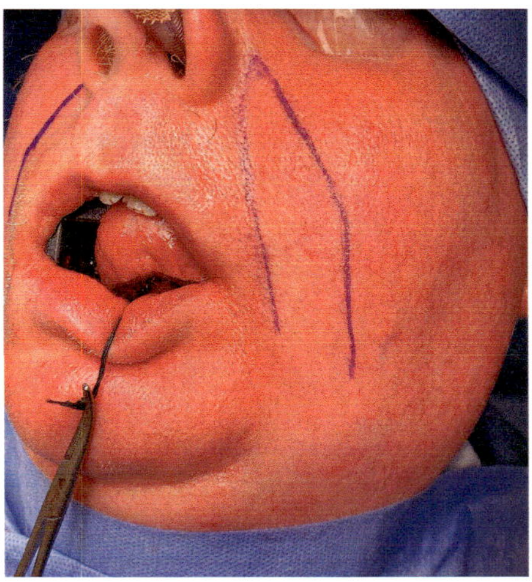

FIGURE 5.6 Pre-operative markings for a nasolabial flap.

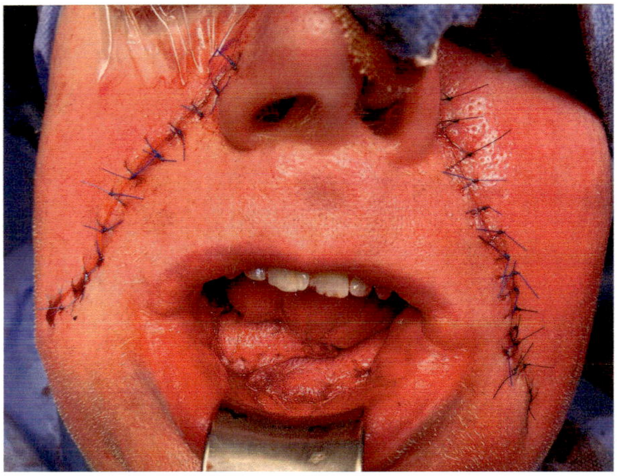

FIGURE 5.7 Flap inset.

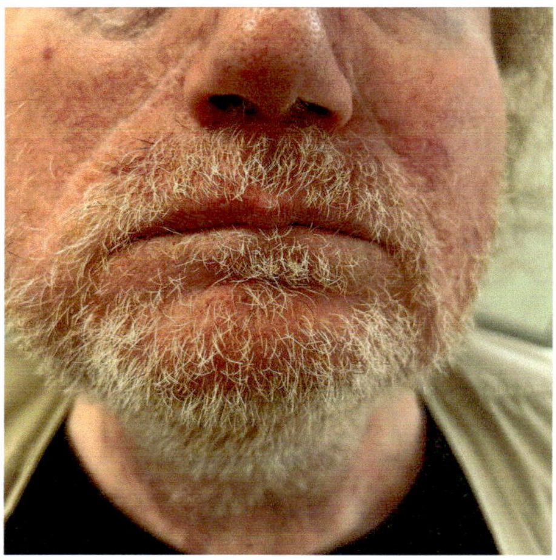

FIGURE 5.8 One-year post-operative scar.

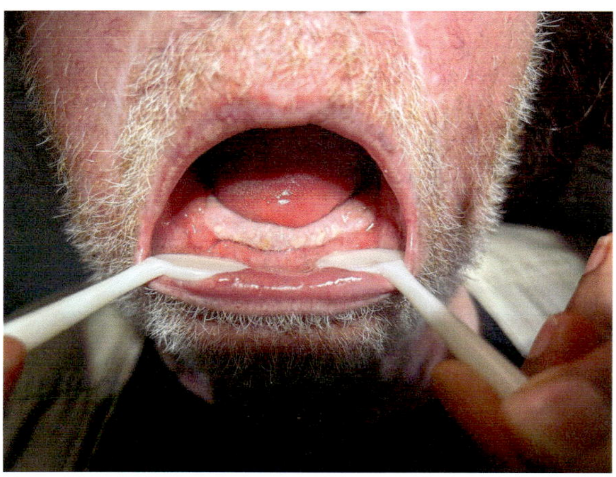

FIGURE 5.9 Intra-oral healing.

Case 5.3

A 65-year-old female who presented with a sublingual gland swelling (low-grade MEC) underwent wide local excision and neck dissection with reconstruction with a nasolabial flap (Figures 5.10 and 5.11).

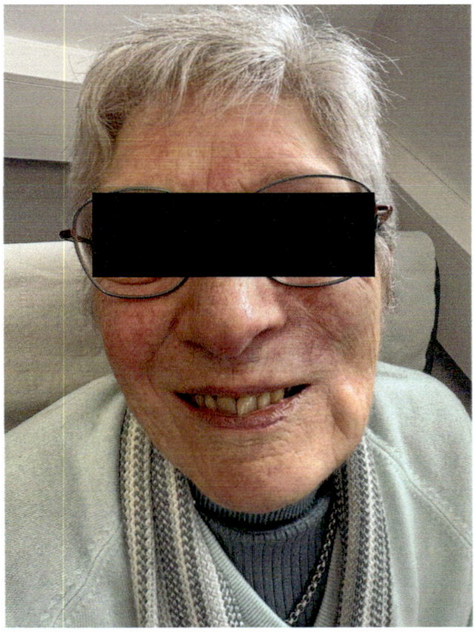

FIGURE 5.10 One-year post-operative left nasolabial flap.

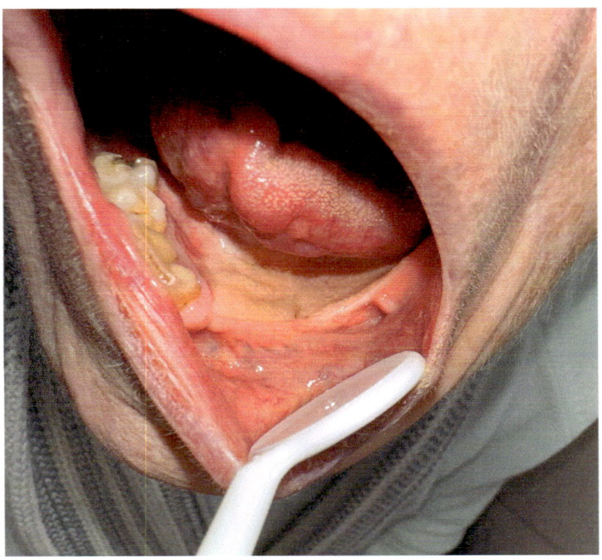

FIGURE 5.11 Left FOM defect after one year.

Case 5.4

A 52-year-old male diagnosed with well-differentiated SCC involving FOM presented to the clinic. The scans showed involvement of underlying muscle and adjacent bone. Wide local excision was performed, followed by placement of a white head varnish pack for 2 weeks. The final histology was pT3N0. The tongue showed good mobility (Figures 5.12–5.17).

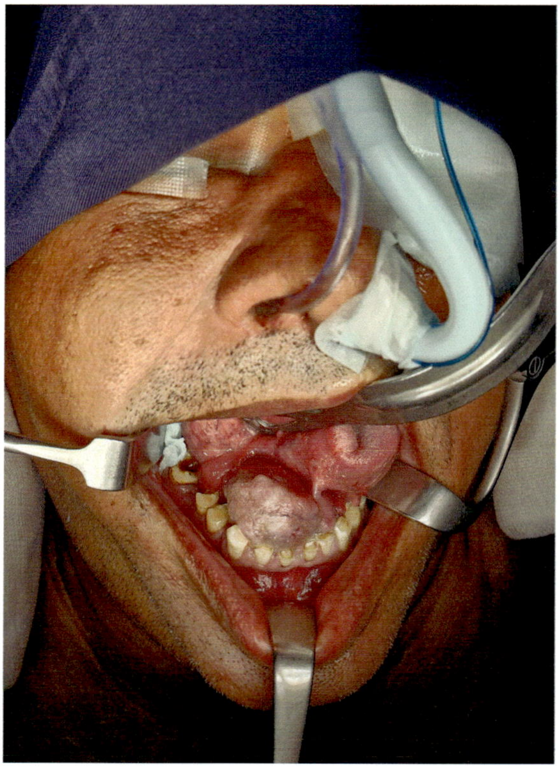

FIGURE 5.12 3 × 2.5 cm exophytic lesion at FOM with no mobility.

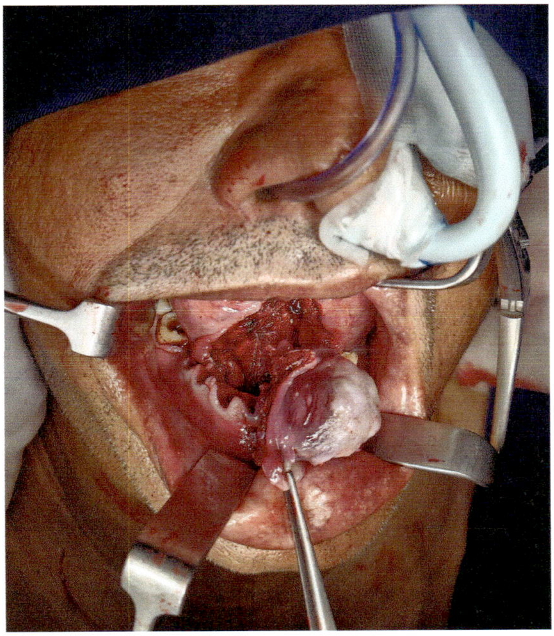

FIGURE 5.13 Intact underlying muscle. The lingual gingiva was removed as part of a soft tissue surgical margin.

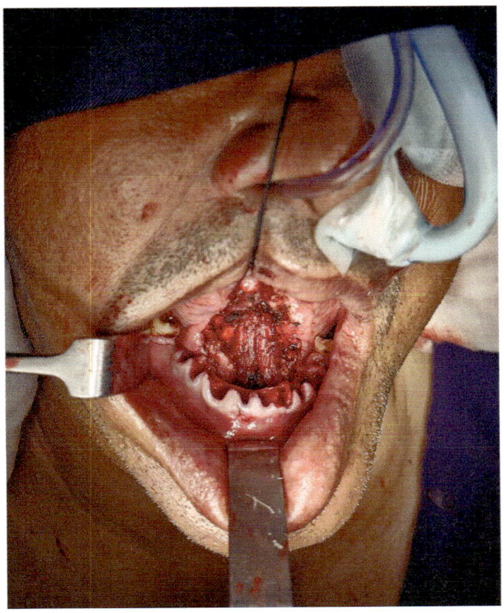

FIGURE 5.14 The surgical bed post-resection showing intact FOM muscles and lower alveolus bone.

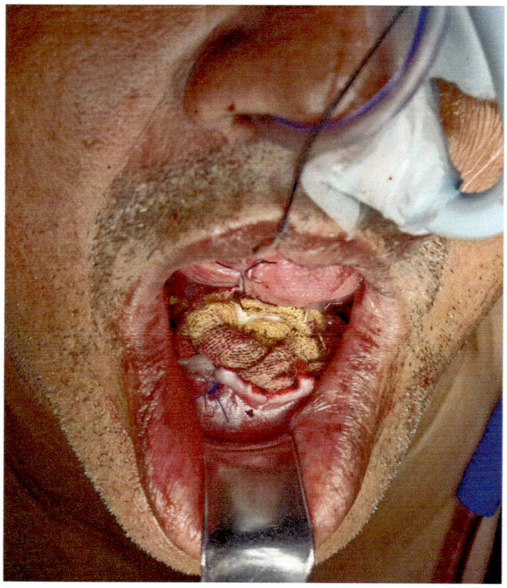

FIGURE 5.15 White head varnish pack sutured in place using a Prolene 3-0 suture.

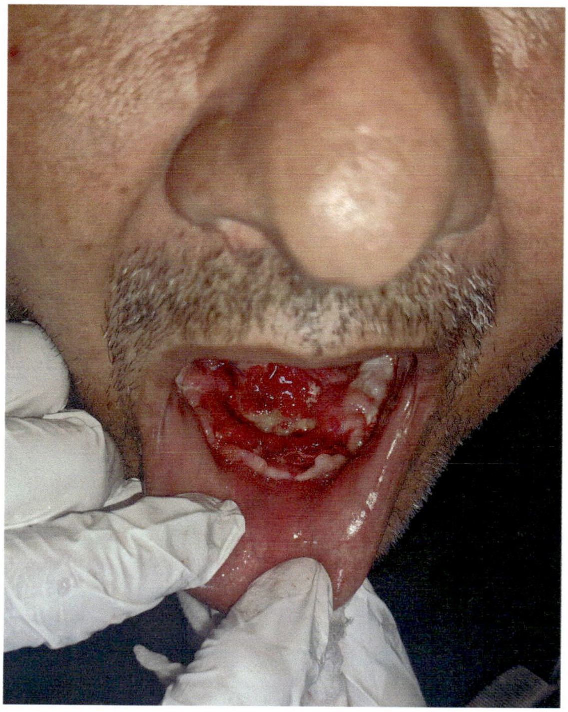

FIGURE 5.16 Day 14 post-operative: White head varnish pack removed, and granulating wound can be appreciated.

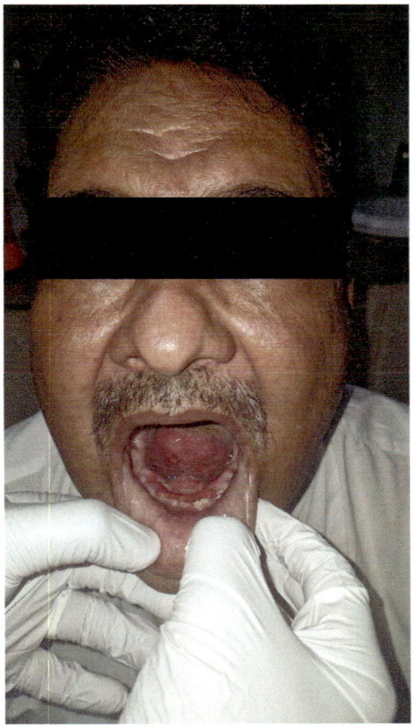

FIGURE 5.17 Day 26 post-operative: Wound is well-healed.

Case 5.5

A patient with left FOM and tongue SCC underwent wide local excision and reconstruction with an FAMM flap. The flap was fully mobilized on its pedicle and reconstructed medial to the mandible to allow for greater rotation of the flap (Figures 5.18–5.21).

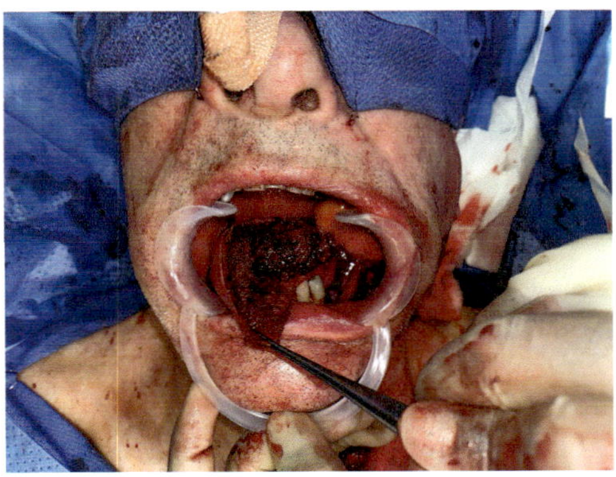

FIGURE 5.18 Resection of the tumor.

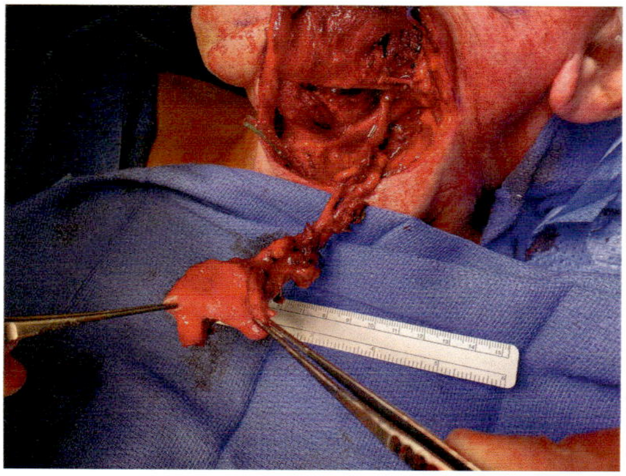

FIGURE 5.19 The FAMM flap on its pedicle.

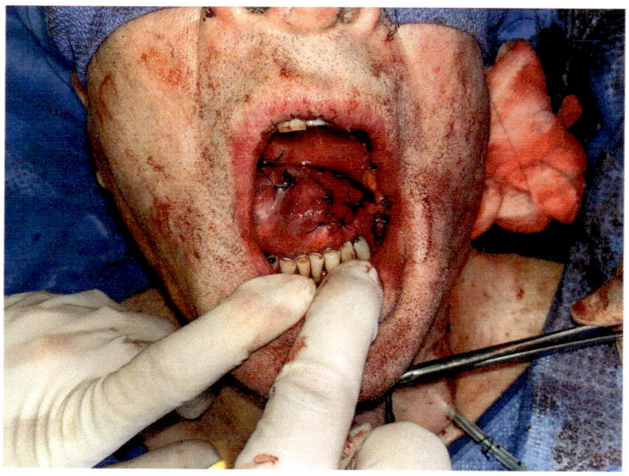

FIGURE 5.20 Flap inset.

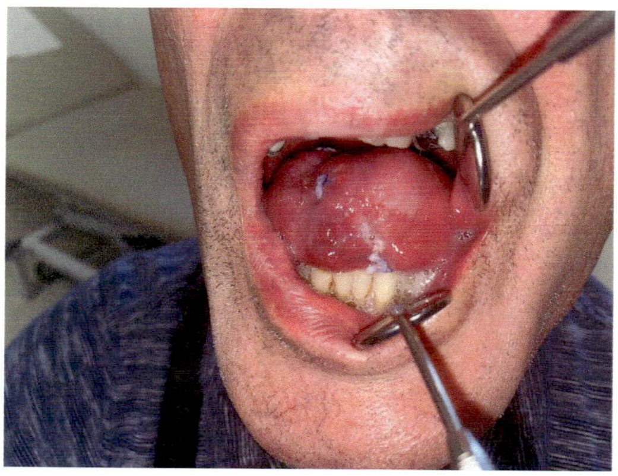

FIGURE 5.21 Four weeks post-operative.

Case 5.6

A 55-year-old female with a small T1 SCC in the right FOM underwent wide local excision, duct transposition, and sentinel node biopsy (Figures 5.22–5.25).

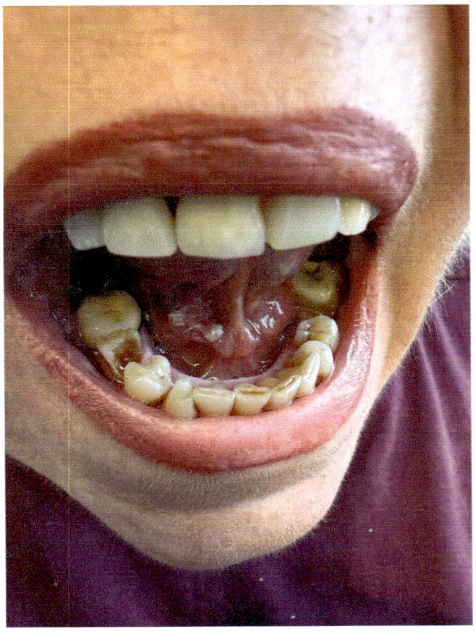

FIGURE 5.22 T1 SCC in the right anterior FOM.

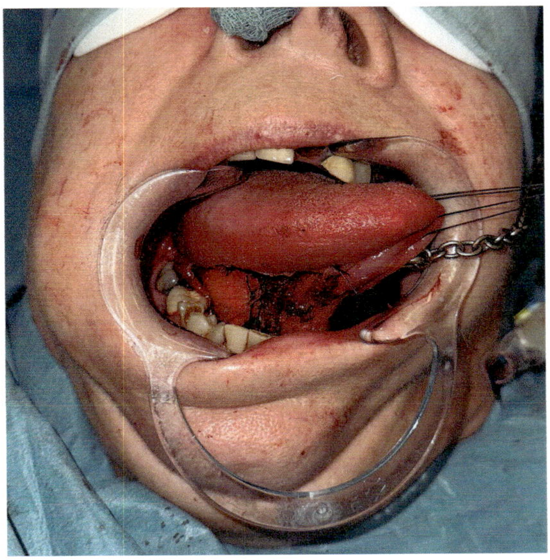

FIGURE 5.23 Wide local excision, local sublingual flap, and then a white head varnish pack.

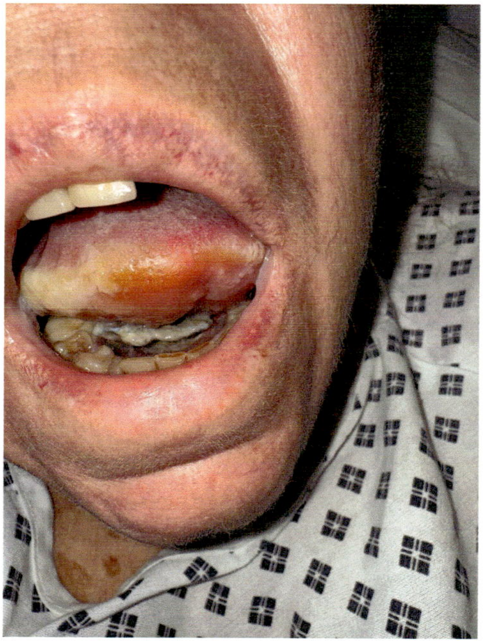

FIGURE 5.24 Four days post-operative. Some tongue edema.

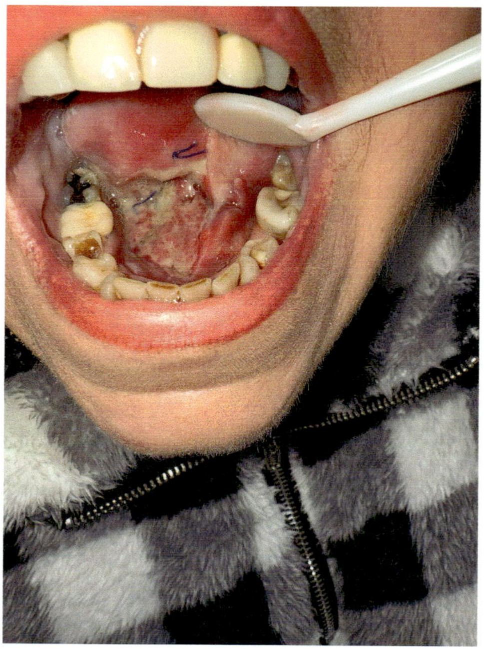

FIGURE 5.25 Two weeks post-operative.

Case 5.7

An elderly female with SCC in the left FOM underwent lip split, mandibulotomy, and reconstruction with a pectoralis major flap (Figures 5.26–5.29).

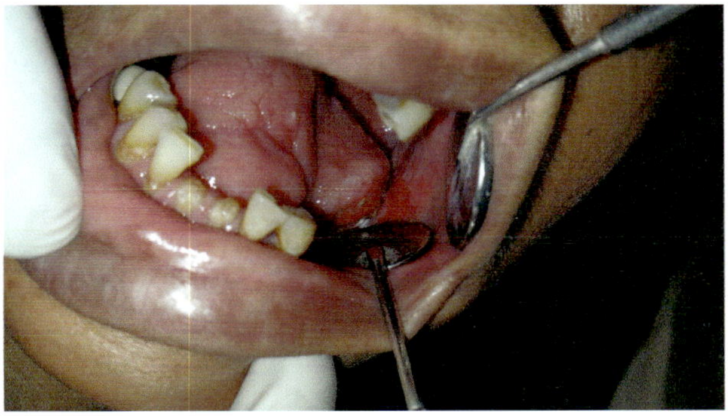

FIGURE 5.26 SCC in the left FOM.

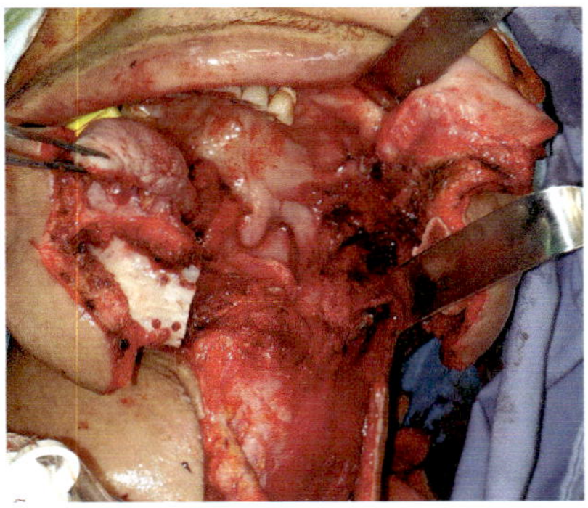

FIGURE 5.27 Lip split and mandibulotomy for access.

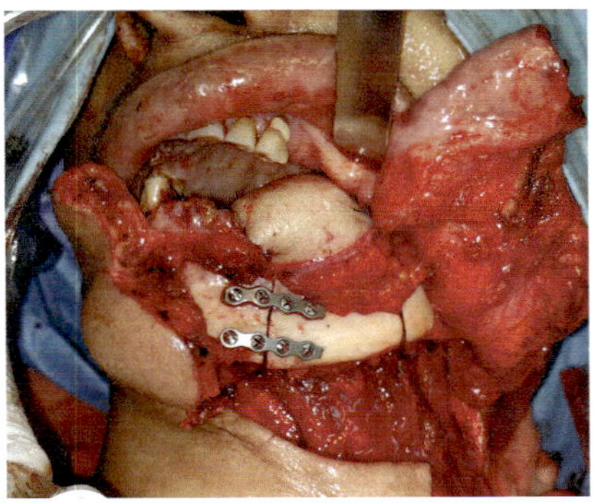

FIGURE 5.28 Pectoralis major flap inset.

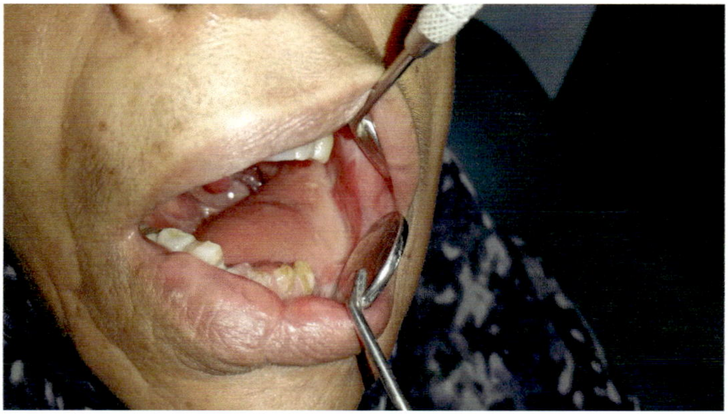

FIGURE 5.29 Several months post-operative.

Case 5.8

A 50-year-old patient with left FOM SCC with alveolus. The patient underwent wide local excision and reconstruction with a deltopectoral (DP) flap (Figures 5.30–5.34).

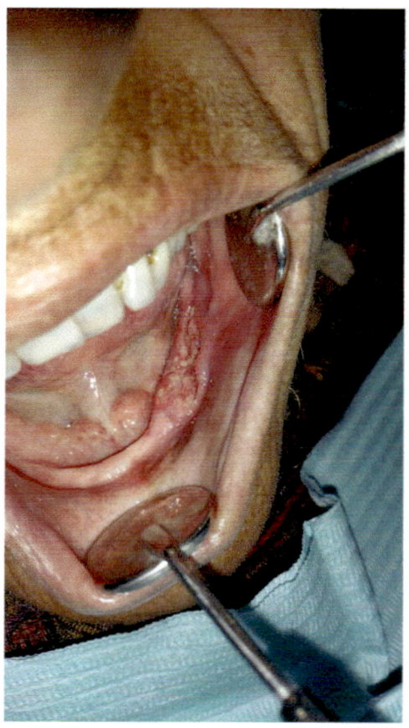

FIGURE 5.30 SCC in the left FOM and attached gingiva.

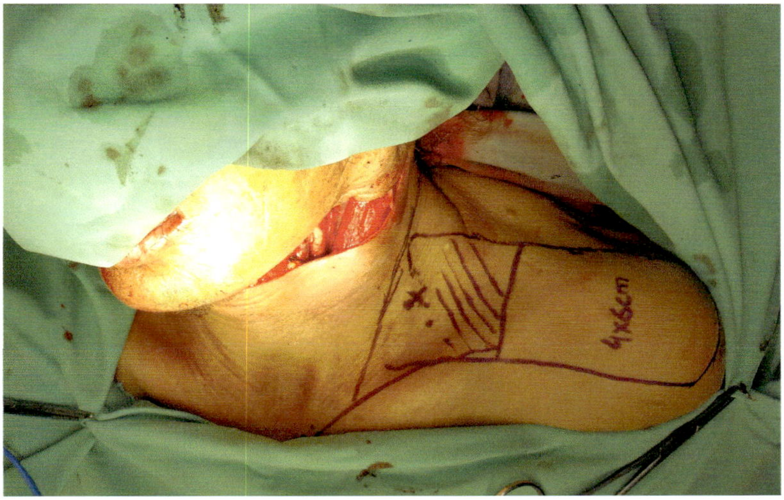

FIGURE 5.31 Markings for a DP flap.

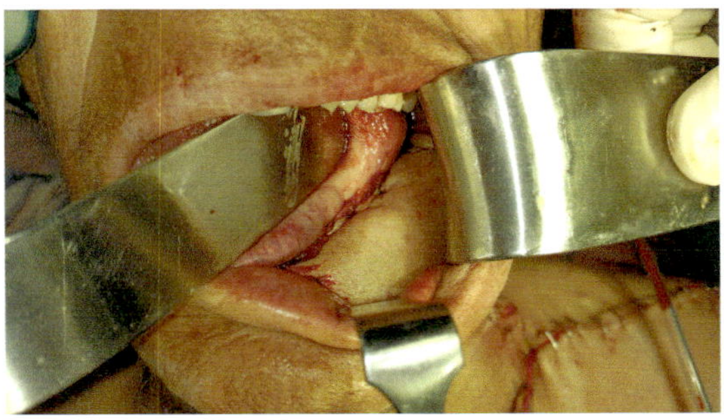

FIGURE 5.32 Flap inset.

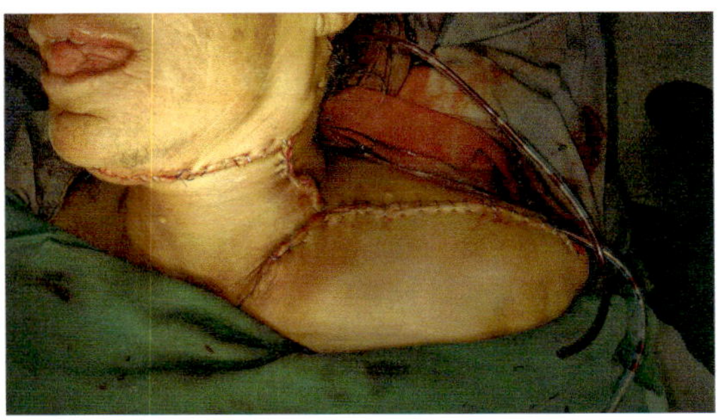

FIGURE 5.33 Closure of the donor site.

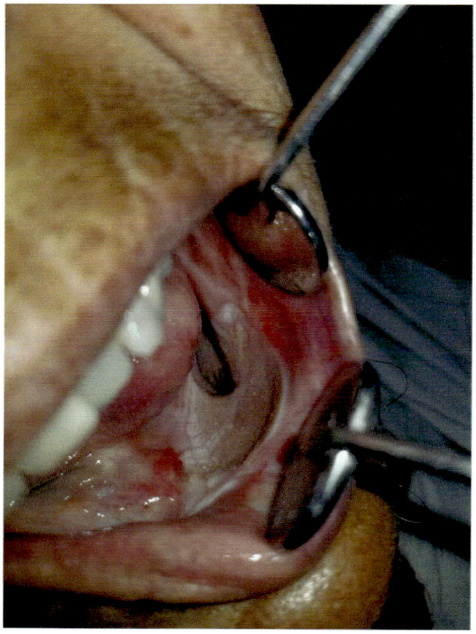

FIGURE 5.34 Several months post-operative.

DISCUSSION

FOM tumors represent a challenging subset of oral cancers due to the region's anatomical complexity and its critical role in speech, swallowing, and oral hygiene. Tumors in this area frequently exhibit aggressive local behavior and are often associated with higher rates of regional metastasis. The management of FOM cancers involves surgical resection, often combined with neck dissection and post-operative radiotherapy, aiming to achieve oncologic control while preserving as much functionality as possible.

- **Anatomy**: The FOM is a small, confined area bordered by the mandible, tongue, and mylohyoid muscle. The close proximity of vital structures, such as the lingual and hypoglossal nerves, salivary ducts, and blood vessels, requires precise surgical technique.
- **Tumor Behavior**: Due to the thin mucosal lining and minimal submucosal tissue, FOM tumors often invade adjacent structures early, such as the mandible and deep tongue musculature, increasing the complexity of achieving clear margins.

- **Wide Local Excision vs. Partial Mandibulectomy**: A major controversy lies in the extent of resection required to achieve negative margins. While some argue that a wide local excision is sufficient for certain early-stage tumors, others advocate for partial mandibulectomy in cases where the tumor approaches or invades the mandible to ensure comprehensive removal. The authors sometimes take the lingual plate as the margin if no bony invasion is noted on the CT scans but clinically it is stuck down at the lingual plate.
- **Close vs. Negative Margins**: The necessity for wide clear margins is widely accepted; however, achieving these in the FOM can be challenging due to anatomical constraints. There is ongoing debate over what constitutes an "adequate" margin in this region, with the mandible abutting and the mylohyoid providing anatomical boundaries.
- **Use of Frozen Section Analysis**: Some surgeons utilize intra-operative frozen sections to confirm margin status, while others argue it adds limited value given the high recurrence rates in this area despite clear margins.
- **Local vs. Free Flaps**: Reconstruction following FOM resection is essential for restoring function and aesthetics. Smaller defects may be addressed with local flaps such as the buccal fat pad or nasolabial flap. However, for extensive resections, free flaps (e.g., a radial forearm or anterolateral thigh flap) are often required to provide sufficient tissue volume and maintain tongue mobility.
- **Elective Neck Dissection**: The authors advocate for routine neck dissection due to the high likelihood of occult metastasis. The authors also routinely do bilateral neck dissections especially close to the midline due to the risk of lymphatic spread. Very small tumors could be considered for sentinel node surgery.
- **Radiotherapy vs. Surgery**: In cases of advanced disease or high nodal burden, the decision between surgery and radiotherapy for managing the neck is controversial. Radiotherapy alone is sometimes preferred to reduce morbidity, though it may compromise regional control. Post-operative radiotherapy is commonly recommended for advanced tumors or those with high-risk features (e.g., positive margins or nodal involvement). However, there is debate over the ideal

dosage and timing, especially in light of the increased risk of complications like osteoradionecrosis when treating tumors adjacent to the mandible.

- **Impact on Speech and Swallowing**: FOM tumors can severely impact oral functions. Reconstructive choices directly influence post-operative speech and swallowing ability, making it essential to balance oncologic success with quality-of-life considerations. Post-operative physiotherapy, speech therapy, and dietary modifications are essential for recovery. Dentures can be difficult to fashion due to lack of sulcus.

CHAPTER 6

Reconstructive Techniques

KEY POINTS

- Discuss various local and regional flaps.
- Anatomy and raising techniques are described.
- Use the QR code to see the videos online.

SUBMENTAL FLAP

The submental flap is a versatile and reliable option for head and neck reconstruction. It utilizes tissue from the submental region (under the chin) to repair defects in areas such as the oral cavity, lower face, and neck. First described in 1993, this flap has gained popularity due to its simplicity, minimal donor site morbidity, and the ease with which it can be harvested. Here, we discuss the key steps involved in raising a submental flap, as well as its advantages and potential complications.

Anatomy

The submental flap is based on the submental artery, which is a branch of the facial artery. The flap can include skin, subcutaneous fat, and platysma muscle, making it ideal for covering various defects, especially those in

DOI: 10.1201/9781032714585-6

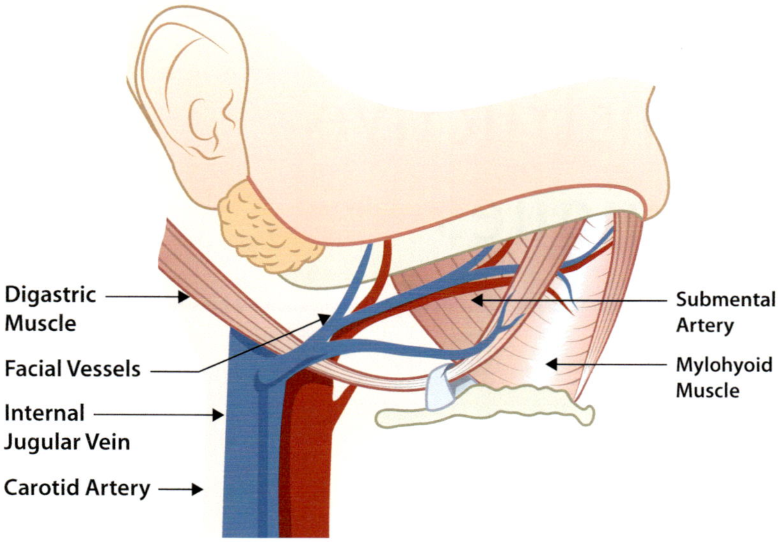

FIGURE 6.1 Anatomy of the submental and submandibular space.

soft tissue. The submental artery runs under the mandible and supplies the tissues of the anterior neck and chin, providing robust vascularization for the flap (Figure 6.1).

Indications for Use

The submental flap is particularly useful in reconstructive surgery for defects following oncologic resection, trauma, or congenital deformities. Common applications include reconstruction of the tongue, floor of the mouth, buccal mucosa, lower lip, and mandibular region. It is favored for moderate-sized defects where free flap reconstruction might be excessive or impractical.

Procedure Overview

- A curvilinear incision is made along the submental crease, which not only hides the scar but also facilitates flap elevation. The upper incision is marked at the level of the inferior border of the mandible from angle to angle, while the lower incision is the limit of the pinch test allowing primary closure adequately (Figure 6.2).
- The lower neck subplatysmal flap is raised first and up to the clavicle to allow adequate traction facilitating primary closure. The upper

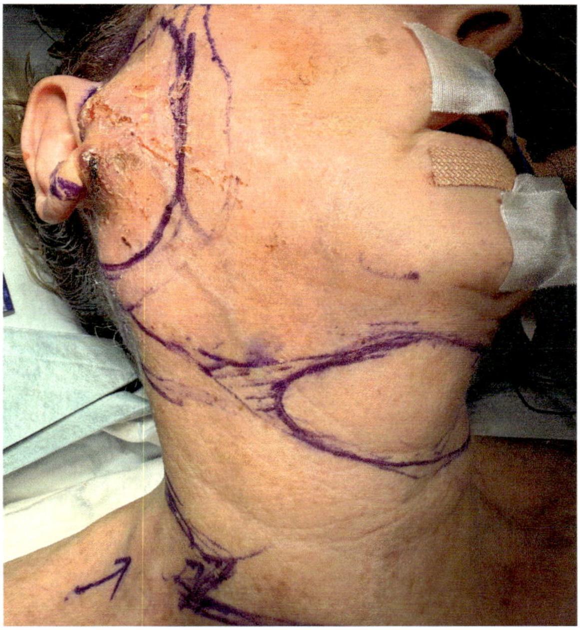

FIGURE 6.2 Skin markings and area to be reconstructed.

cervical flap is raised afterward while carefully identifying and protecting the marginal mandibular nerve.

- The subplatysmal dissection is performed adjacent to the inferior border of the mandible anteriorly including the ipsilateral anterior belly of the digastric muscle. While raising the flap, platysma is sutured to the skin paddle to protect cutaneous perforators.
- The contralateral side of the flap is raised up to the midline in the subplatysmal plane. The facial vessel above the origin of the submental vessel needs to be ligated when using a proximally based flap.
- The submandibular gland is carefully dissected off the facial vessels while identifying and ligating the glandular branches.
- The facial vein has quite a variable course draining either directly into internal jugular vein or external jugular vein by communicating with the facial vein and anterior division of the retromandibular vein.
- Once the submental artery and vein are identified, the flap is raised in a pedicled fashion. This ensures that the blood supply remains intact during transposition (Figure 6.3).

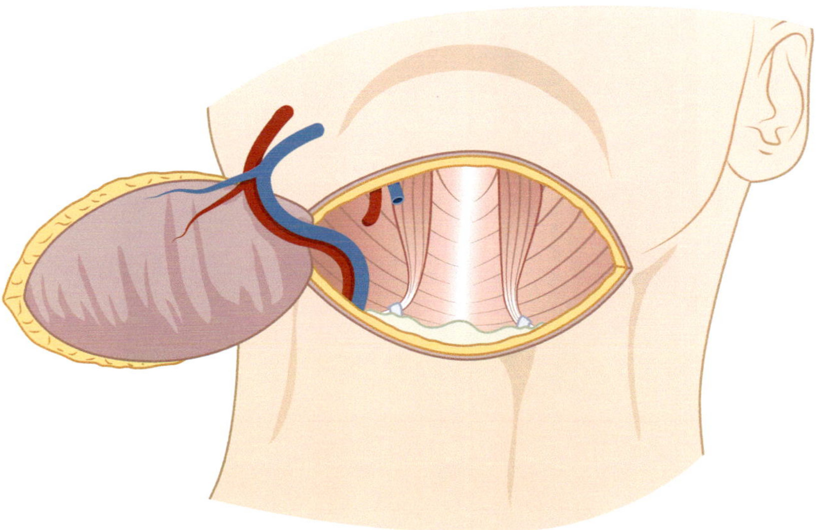

FIGURE 6.3 Facial artery and facial vein with platysma muscle.

- Depending on the size of the defect, the flap can include skin, subcutaneous tissue, and muscle. The pedicle is long enough to allow the flap to reach various parts of the head and neck without tension.
- The donor site is closed primarily, provided the tissue harvested does not cause significant tension.

Advantages

The submental flap has several advantages:

- **Minimal Donor Site Morbidity**: Since the donor site is easily concealed and can often be closed primarily; the aesthetic outcomes are favorable.
- **Ease of Harvesting**: The flap is relatively simple to raise and does not require microvascular anastomosis.
- **Versatility**: The flap can be used to cover a range of defects in the oral cavity, neck, and lower face.
- **Good Aesthetic Outcomes**: The donor site scar is hidden under the chin, making it cosmetically acceptable.

Potential Complications

As with any flap, complications such as flap ischemia, necrosis, or infection can occur. Venous congestion is a potential issue due to the pedicled nature of the flap, and careful intra-operative technique is required to minimize this risk. Additionally, some patients may experience discomfort or numbness in the submental region after the procedure.

There is an ongoing controversy and debate about the oncological safety and potential risk of occult disease transfer to the recipient site while using this flap.

The flap has a good arc of rotation covering the whole homolateral face and the oral cavity, except for a part of the forehead.

The flap has a very predictable arterial course, but the venous drainage has minor variations sufficient to surprise the operating surgeon. The venous drainage can be into the internal jugular vein, the external jugular vein, and at times into the anterior jugular vein.

Conclusion

The submental flap is an effective and reliable option for reconstructing moderate defects in the head and neck region. Its ease of harvest, favorable aesthetic outcomes, and robust blood supply make it a preferred choice for surgeons in select cases. However, careful patient selection, meticulous technique, and post-operative care are crucial for optimal outcomes.

TEMPORALIS FLAP

The temporalis muscle flap is a versatile option that has been employed successfully to reconstruct various defects within the oral cavity. We discuss the anatomy, indications, surgical technique, advantages, limitations, and post-operative considerations associated with the use of the temporalis flap in oral cavity cancer reconstruction.

Anatomy

The temporalis muscle is a broad, fan-shaped muscle located on the lateral side of the skull. It originates from the temporal fossa and the temporal fascia and inserts onto the coronoid process of the mandible. The muscle is innervated by the deep temporal branches of the mandibular nerve (cranial nerve V3) and receives its blood supply primarily from the deep temporal arteries, branches of the maxillary artery (Figure 6.4).

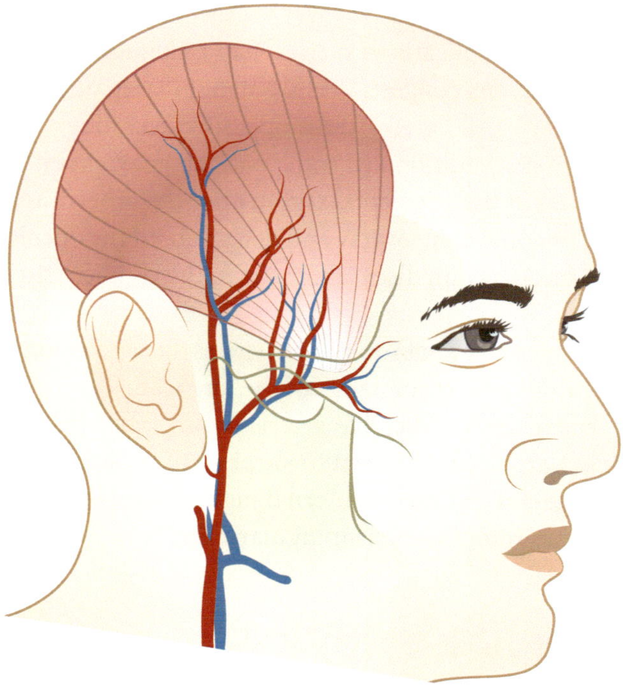

FIGURE 6.4 Anatomy of the temporalis flap.

Understanding the anatomy is crucial for flap elevation. The muscle is covered by a robust fascia, which can be included in the flap to enhance its reach and versatility. The proximity of the temporalis muscle to the oral cavity makes it an excellent option for reconstruction without the need for microvascular anastomosis.

Indications for Use

The temporalis flap is indicated in the reconstruction of moderate to large defects of the oral cavity, particularly when other local or regional flaps are not suitable. Specific indications include:

- Reconstruction of defects of the maxilla, palate, cheek, and retromolar trigone.
- Cases where previous radiation therapy limits the use of other flaps.
- Patients unsuitable for free flap surgery due to comorbidities or lack of microsurgical facilities.

Procedure Overview

- **Incision**: A hemi-coronal or linear incision is made above the zygomatic arch to expose the temporalis muscle. The incision is marked from the pre-auricular area and then runs along the superior aspect of the helical rim, turning toward the superior temporal line and stopping within the hairline anteriorly. Incision is placed along the marked line, keeping the depth up to the dermis in the pre-auricular area and the temporoparietal fascia in the scalp area (Figure 6.5).
    - The anterior and posterior scalp flaps are elevated, and the temporalis muscle with its fan-shaped presence is easily identified (Figure 6.6).
    - An anterior incision over the fascia is placed by respecting the Pitanguy's line running from 0.5 cm below the tragus and 1.5 cm above the lateral eyebrow to avoid injury to the frontal branch of the facial nerve. Once the dissection reaches the pre-auricular area close to the insertion of muscle to the coronoid process and anterior ramus border, one must be careful to avoid injuring the deep temporal vessels (Figure 6.7).

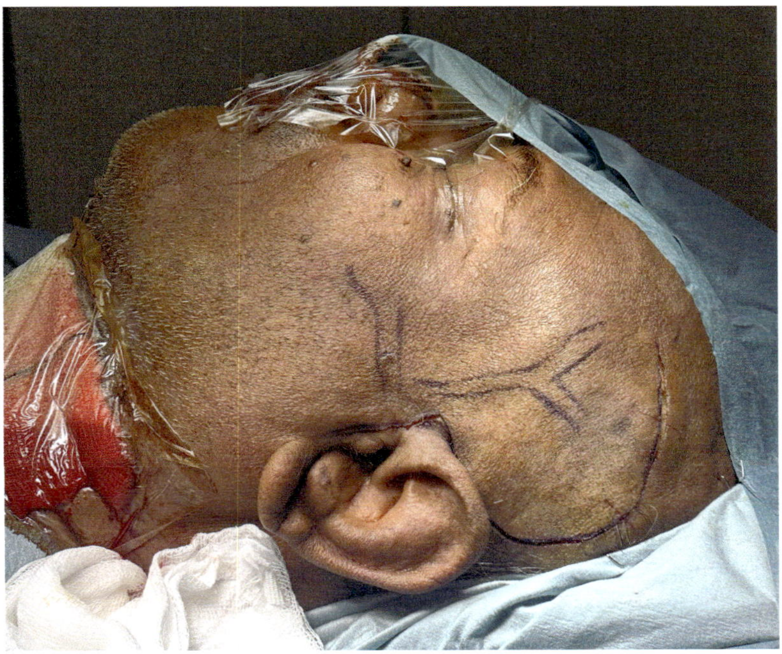

FIGURE 6.5 Marking of incision and vasculature.

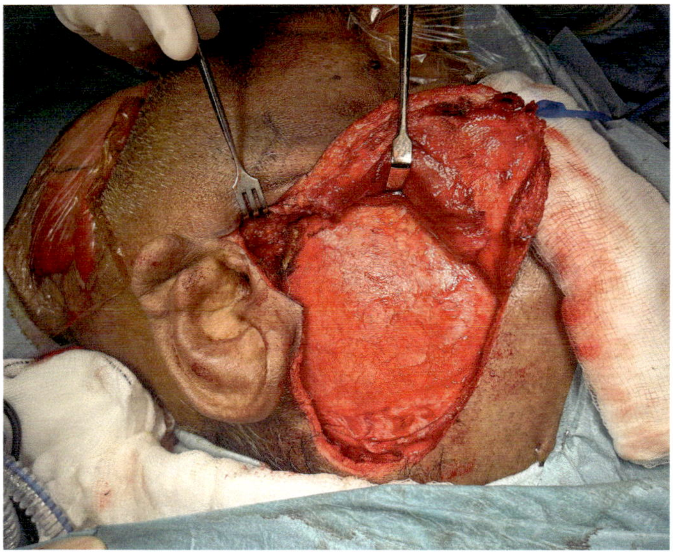

FIGURE 6.6 Temporalis flap raised above the temporal bone.

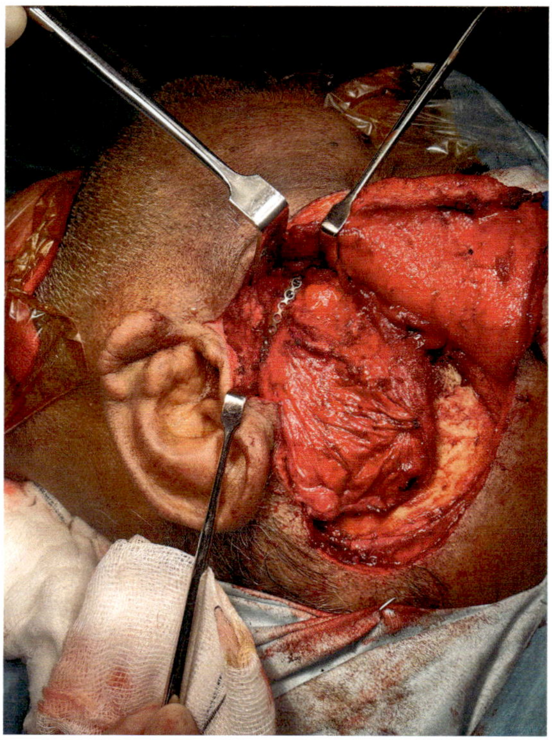

FIGURE 6.7 Flap raised and zygomatic arch pre-plated prior to osteotomy.

- Depending upon the requirement of the muscle, one can start elevating the muscle anteroposteriorly above the bone in the inferior direction. The muscle can be harvested along the temporoparietal fascia, resulting in fascial covering and less bleeding post-operatively.

- **Flap Rotation**: The muscle is passed through a tunnel created in the zygomatic arch or around it to reach the oral cavity defect. The muscle can be brought into the oral cavity by two approaches (Figure 6.8):
  - Under the zygomatic arch, which sometimes needs osteotomy.
  - Over the zygomatic arch but with decreased reach.
- **Insetting the Flap**: The muscle is shaped to fit the defect and secured in place with sutures.
- **Donor Site Closure**: The temporal fascia is closed, and the scalp incision is sutured in layers.

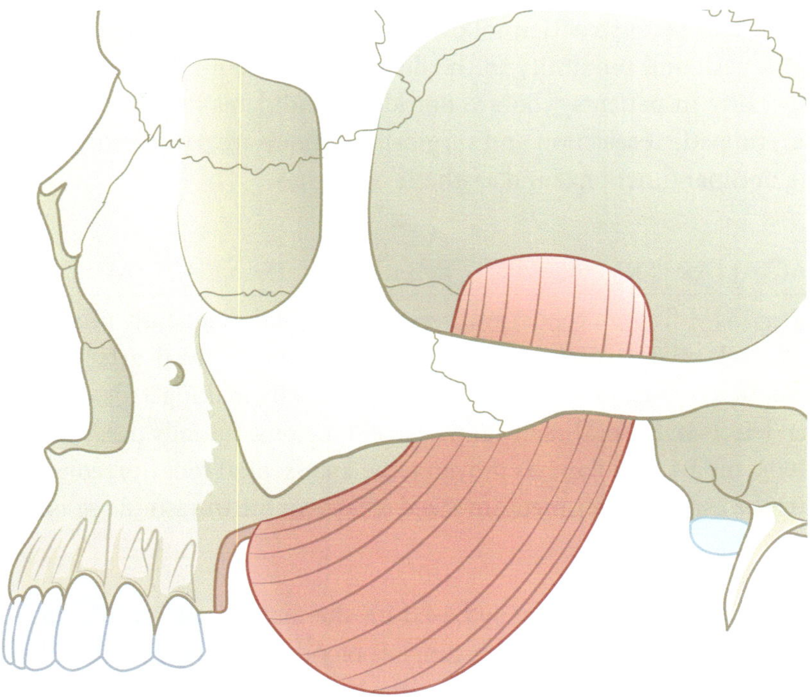

FIGURE 6.8 Flap brought into the oral cavity below the zygomatic arch.

Advantages

- **Proximity**: Close to the oral cavity, allowing for quick transfer without microvascular anastomosis.
- **Reliability**: Robust blood supply ensures high flap survival rates.
- **Versatility**: Can be modified to suit various defect sizes and shapes.
- **Reduced Operating Time**: Faster than free flap procedures.

Potential Complications

- **Donor Site Morbidity**: Potential for temporal hollowing and mandibular dysfunction.
- **Limited Reach**: May not be suitable for defects distant from the muscle's arc of rotation.
- **Bulkiness**: May result in over-contouring, requiring secondary revisions.

Conclusion

The temporalis flap remains a valuable tool in the armamentarium for oral cavity reconstruction following cancer resection. Its reliability, ease of harvest, and proximity to the defect site make it an attractive option, especially in patients who are not ideal candidates for free flap surgery. Careful patient selection and surgical technique are paramount to achieving optimal functional and aesthetic outcomes.

FACIAL ARTERY MUSCULOMUCOSAL (FAMM) FLAP

The FAMM flap is a robust and versatile local flap frequently used for head and neck reconstruction. This flap, based on the facial artery, includes mucosa, submucosa, muscle, and sometimes skin, making it ideal for repairing defects in the oral cavity and adjacent regions. Initially described in the 1990s, the FAMM flap has proven to be an essential tool in reconstructive surgery, especially for medium-sized defects in the intra-oral region.

Anatomy

The FAMM flap is primarily based on the facial artery, a branch of the external carotid artery, which supplies blood to the flap. The facial artery courses across the mandible, along the buccinator muscle, and it provides robust vascular support to the flap. This flap incorporates layers of mucosa, submucosa, and muscle, making it particularly suited for intra-oral reconstructions (Figure 6.9).

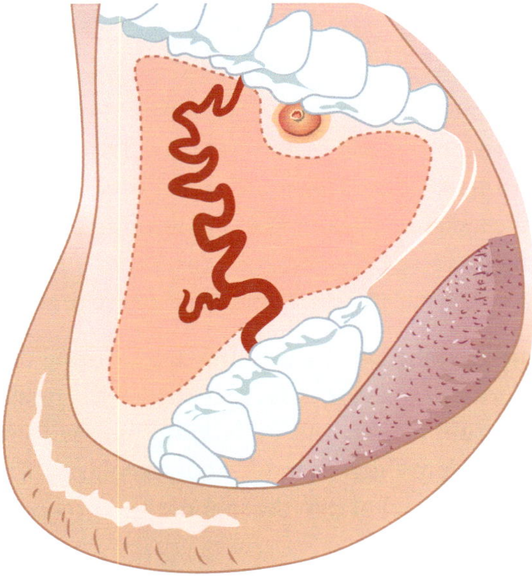

FIGURE 6.9 FAMM flap anatomy.

There are two main types of FAMM flaps based on the orientation of the pedicle:

- **Superiorly Based FAMM Flap**: Uses the distal portion of the facial artery, making it suitable for defects located higher in the oral cavity, such as the palate, upper lip, and hard palate.
- **Inferiorly Based FAMM Flap**: Utilizes the proximal facial artery, making it ideal for lower intra-oral defects like the floor of the mouth, lower lip, and mandibular region.

Indications for Use

The FAMM flap is particularly valuable for reconstructing soft tissue defects within the oral cavity, such as those resulting from oncologic resection, trauma, or congenital conditions. Common sites of reconstruction include:

- Oral mucosal defects
- Palatal and buccal defects
- Lip reconstruction
- Floor of the mouth
- Alveolar ridge and tongue

Procedure Overview

- The incision is made along the buccal mucosa, typically following the anatomic course of the facial artery. For a superiorly based flap, the incision is made higher in the oral cavity, while for an inferiorly based flap, it starts lower. Careful dissection is performed to preserve the facial artery and the surrounding musculo-mucosal tissue. During this stage, the surgeon must avoid injuring critical structures such as the parotid duct and facial nerve branches.
- After identifying the facial artery and determining the pedicle orientation (superior or inferior), the flap is elevated. The surgeon includes the mucosa, submucosa, and underlying muscle (typically the buccinator), which provides strength and vascularity. The flap remains pedicled on the facial artery throughout the procedure to maintain perfusion.
- Once the flap is raised, it is rotated or advanced to cover the defect in the oral cavity or facial region. Its flexibility allows it to be used for defects in the lips, floor of the mouth, or even the hard palate. The flap is inset into the defect with careful suturing to minimize tension. The donor site is typically closed primarily, although the buccal fat pad can be used if the defect is too large to close directly.
- For dentate patients the flap can be raised on its pedicle and brought out into the neck. This can then subsequently be tunneled medial to the mandible for insetting (Figure 6.10).

Advantages

The FAMM flap offers several distinct advantages:

- **Good Functional and Aesthetic Outcomes**: The FAMM flap provides an excellent tissue match in terms of color, texture, and functionality. Since it is harvested from the mucosa, it is ideal for intra-oral repairs and blends well with the surrounding tissues.
- **Ease of Harvesting**: The flap is relatively easy to raise, requiring no microvascular anastomosis, which simplifies the procedure.
- **Flexibility**: The flap can be used to cover a variety of defects in both the upper and lower oral cavity, making it versatile for different types of reconstruction.

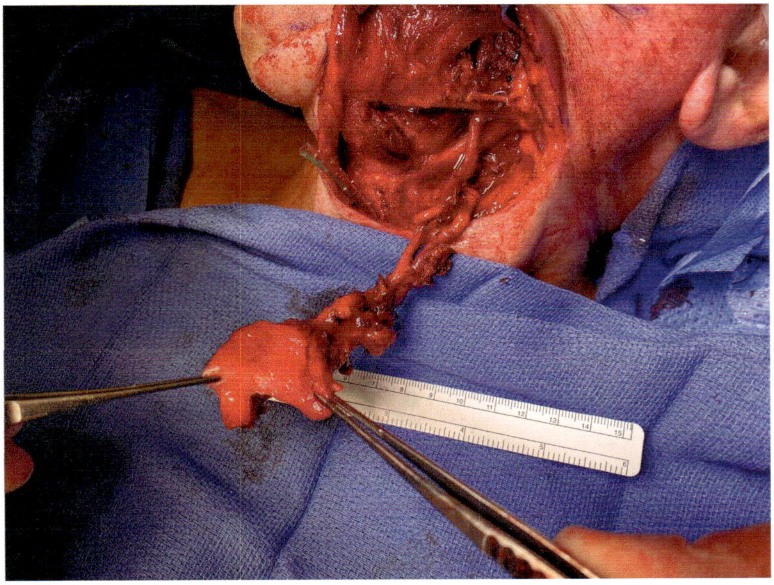

FIGURE 6.10 FAMM flap brought out into the neck to improve the arc of rotation.

- **Minimal Donor Site Morbidity**: The donor site is inside the oral cavity, leading to minimal visible scarring and a concealed donor site, making it cosmetically favorable.

Potential Complications

As with any surgical procedure, the FAMM flap has some risks. Venous congestion and partial flap necrosis are the most common complications due to the flap's pedicled nature. Surgeons must be vigilant about preserving the vascular pedicle to minimize these risks. Other potential issues include infection, wound dehiscence, and, in rare cases, damage to adjacent structures such as the parotid duct or facial nerve branches. Donor site complications, though rare, may include intra-oral scarring or trismus. This can be alleviated with buccal fat pad donor site repair.

Conclusion

The FAMM flap is an effective and reliable technique for reconstructing soft tissue defects in the oral cavity and adjacent regions. Its robust blood supply, versatility, and ability to be harvested from the oral cavity with minimal donor site morbidity make it a preferred option in head and neck reconstruction. Careful surgical planning and technique are crucial to achieving optimal functional and aesthetic outcomes.

DELTOPECTORAL (DP) FLAP

The DP flap is a reliable and versatile option for reconstructive surgery, particularly in the head and neck region. First introduced in the 1960s, it has remained a valuable choice for covering extensive soft tissue defects. This flap is appreciated for its consistent vascularity, simplicity in design, and applicability to a range of defects.

Anatomy

The DP flap is based on the perforators of the internal thoracic artery or, in some cases, the thoracoacromial artery. It involves skin and subcutaneous tissue from the anterior chest wall, extending from the clavicle to the deltoid region. Its rich vascularity allows for robust healing and reliable coverage of defects in the head, neck (below zygomatic arch), and upper thorax (Figure 6.11).

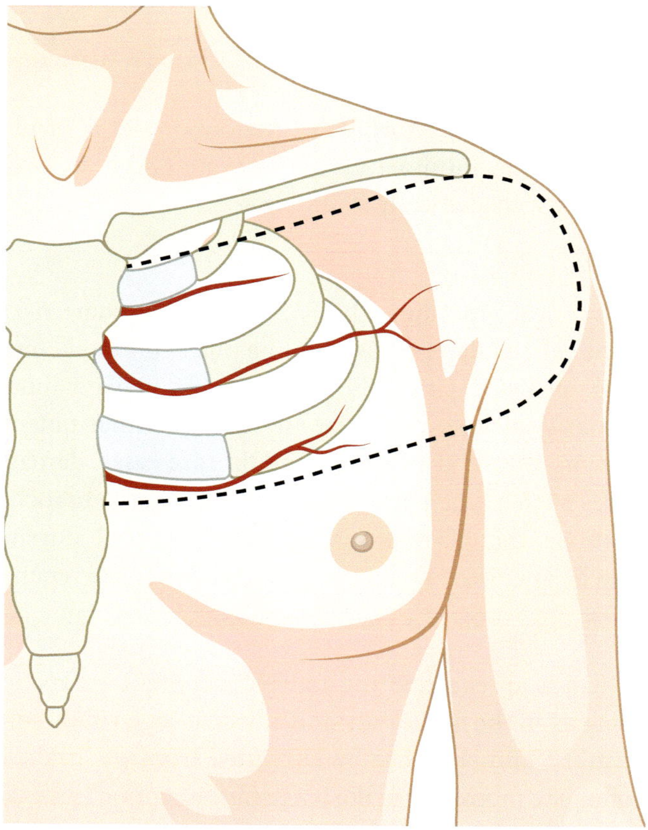

FIGURE 6.11 Anatomy showing medial perforators and skin marking.

Indications for Use

The DP flap is particularly useful in cases requiring reconstruction of large soft tissue defects following:

- Resection of head and neck tumors.
- Repair of pharyngoesophageal or tracheal defects.
- Reconstruction after trauma or congenital deformities.

It is most effective in situations where free flaps may not be feasible due to patient factors or resource limitations.

Procedure Overview

- Identify the boundaries based on defect size and location.
- Use the deltopectoral groove and clavicle as anatomical references for flap orientation.
- Keep the medial edge close to the midline to ensure a robust blood supply from the perforators of the internal thoracic artery.
- Incise along the marked lines, extending through the skin and subcutaneous tissue.
- Carefully preserve the underlying fascia to maintain vascular supply.
- Begin from the distal end and proceed proximally toward the chest midline.

Identify and preserve the internal thoracic artery perforators at the medial end of the flap. Recommend ultrasound to identify and mark internal mammary perforators.

- Avoid excessive torsion or stretching of the pedicle during mobilization to prevent vascular compromise.
- Rotate or transpose the flap to the recipient site. For defects in the head and neck, route the flap through a subcutaneous tunnel if needed to reduce external scarring.
- Avoid tension on the vascular pedicle during inset.
- Close the donor site primarily if feasible.
- For larger defects, a split-thickness skin graft may be required.

Advantages

- **Robust Vascularity**: Ensures reliable healing, even in irradiated fields.
- **Ease of Harvest**: Does not require microvascular expertise.
- **Wide Applicability**: Covers extensive defects, particularly in the head and neck region.
- **Minimal Donor Morbidity**: The anterior chest provides an inconspicuous donor site.

Potential Complications

- **Flap Ischemia or Necrosis**: May occur if vascular supply is compromised during raising.
- **Donor Site Issues**: Tension or improper closure can lead to scarring or poor healing.
- **Limited Arc of Rotation**: The reach of the flap may be insufficient for distant defects.

Conclusion

The DP flap remains a cornerstone in reconstructive surgery due to its reliability and versatility. While free flaps have gained popularity, the DP flap continues to serve as an essential option in settings where simpler, robust solutions are required. Meticulous technique and careful patient selection ensure optimal outcomes.

PALATAL ISLAND FLAP

The palatal island flap is a versatile and commonly used reconstructive technique for small- to medium-sized defects in the oral cavity, particularly in the palate. It is ideal for defects resulting from oncologic resections, trauma, or congenital deformities.

Anatomy

The palatal island flap is a mucoperiosteal flap based on the greater palatine artery and nerve.

- **Blood Supply**: Primarily the greater palatine artery, a branch of the descending palatine artery, which exits the greater palatine foramen (near the third maxillary molar) and runs anteriorly along the hard palate.

- **Innervation**: The greater palatine nerve accompanies the artery, providing sensation.
- **Composition**: Consists of palatal mucosa and underlying periosteum.
- **Key Feature**: Its axial blood supply allows it to be elevated as an "island" of tissue, maintaining viability while being rotated to reconstruct defects.

Indications for Use

1. **Post-Ablative Defects of the Palate (Hard and/or Soft)**: This is the most common indication. Following surgical removal of benign or malignant lesions (e.g., squamous cell carcinoma, minor salivary gland tumors) from the hard or soft palate, the palatal island flap can be used to:
   - Separate the oral and nasal cavities: Crucial for preventing regurgitation of food/liquids into the nose and maintaining intelligible speech.
   - Restore functional integrity: Helps in speech, swallowing, and breathing.
   - Avoid the need for prosthetic obturation: In many cases, it eliminates the need for a removable prosthesis to cover the palatal defect.
2. **Retromolar Trigone Defects**: The flap's arc of rotation allows it to reach defects in the retromolar trigone (the triangular area behind the last molar tooth), often seen after cancer resection in this area.
3. **Tonsillar Fossa Defects**: Can be used for smaller defects in the tonsillar area.
4. **Limited Defects of the Cheek and Posterior Floor of Mouth**: While less common than palatal reconstruction, its versatility allows for its use in select small to medium-sized defects in these adjacent areas.

Procedure Overview

- Assess the defect's size, location, and orientation to design the flap accordingly.
- The flap is generally pedicled on the greater palatine artery for vascular supply (Figure 6.12).

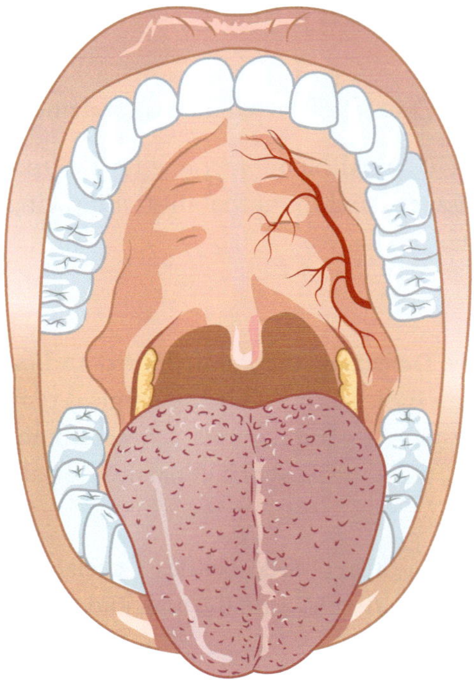

FIGURE 6.12 Anatomy of the palatal island flap.

- Confirm the patient's oral hygiene and condition of the palatal mucosa.
- Using a surgical marker, outline the flap design on the hard palate.
- Make a mucoperiosteal incision using a sharp blade along the marked lines.
- Ensure preservation of the vascular pedicle (greater palatine artery).
- Carefully elevate the mucoperiosteum from the underlying hard palate using a periosteal elevator.
- Begin at the edges and gradually work toward the vascular pedicle.
- Avoid perforation into the nasal cavity to preserve integrity.
- Mobilize the flap by gently stretching it to assess its reach to the defect (Figure 6.13).

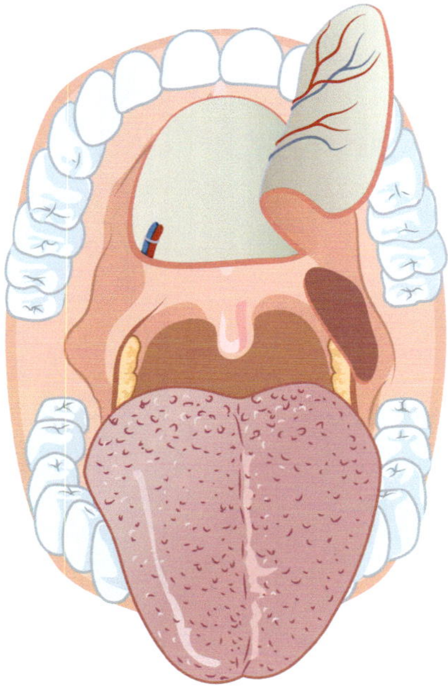

FIGURE 6.13 Flap raised on a pedicle.

- If additional mobility is required, incise the periosteum at strategic points while preserving the pedicle.
- Rotate or advance the flap to the defect site, ensuring no tension on the pedicle.
- Inset the flap and secure it with absorbable sutures (Figure 6.14).
- The donor site is often left to heal by secondary intention or covered with a soft dressing.

Advantages

- Proximity to the defect
- Preserves oral and nasal functions
- Minimal donor site morbidity

Potential Complications

- Donor site pain or scarring
    - Risk of necrosis if vascular supply is compromised

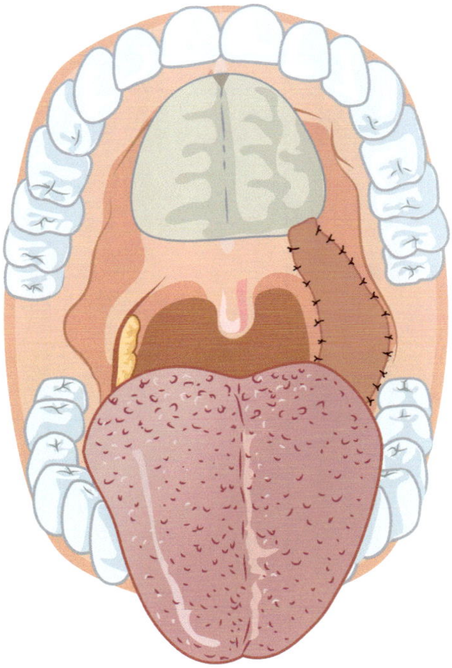

FIGURE 6.14 Flap inset to the defect.

PECTORALIS MAJOR FLAP (PMF)

The PMF is a robust and versatile reconstructive option for defects in the head, neck, and upper chest regions. Since its introduction in the mid-twentieth century, it has been a preferred choice for covering moderate to large defects due to its ease of harvest, reliable vascular supply, and the minimal donor site morbidity it entails. Below is an overview of the anatomy, indications, procedural steps, and advantages associated with this flap.

Anatomy

The PMF is based on the thoracoacromial artery, with possible additional contributions from the lateral thoracic and internal mammary arteries. The flap can include the pectoralis major muscle, skin, and subcutaneous tissue, offering sufficient bulk and flexibility for reconstruction. The thoracoacromial artery's perforators provide robust vascularization, ensuring a dependable blood supply during flap elevation and transfer.

Indications for Use

The PMF is ideal for reconstructive surgery addressing defects caused by:

- Oncologic resection in the head and neck.
- Tracheoesophageal or pharyngocutaneous fistula repair.
- Sternal dehiscence or chest wall trauma.
- Reconstructive surgeries in patients unsuitable for microvascular free flaps.

Its versatility and predictability make it particularly valuable in scenarios where free tissue transfer is not feasible due to patient factors or resource constraints.

Procedure Overview

- The patient is placed supine with the arm abducted to 90° on an armboard. A line is drawn from the medial tip of the coracoid process to the xiphisternum, approximating the course of the thoracoacromial vessels (Figure 6.15). The flap is outlined, taking into consideration the anatomical landmarks of the pectoralis major muscle (Figure 6.15).

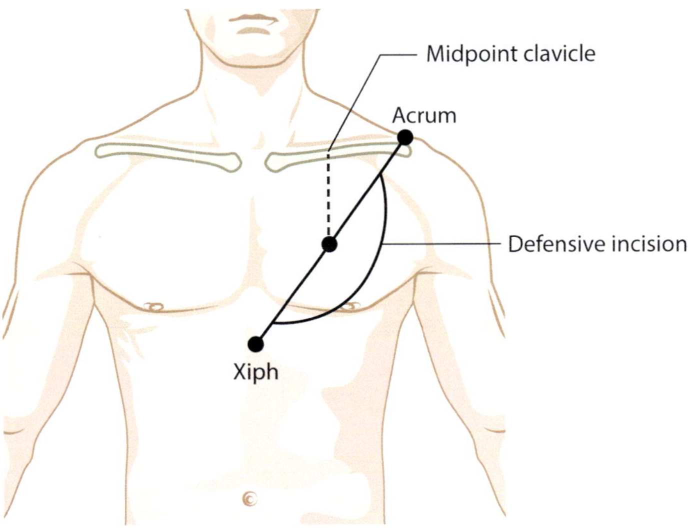

FIGURE 6.15 Identifying the vascular pedicle.

- For males, the skin paddle is designed as an elliptical shape along the pedicle marking. In females, a horizontal sub-mammary incision is preferred to maintain cosmesis. The lower margin of the skin paddle should align with the costal margin, avoiding excessive extension inferiorly to maintain skin viability.
- The skin incision is made along the predefined paddle through the subcutaneous fat to the underlying muscle. Subcutaneous fat along the pedicle is preserved to enhance perforator integrity. The muscle is dissected from the chest wall, working along the rib periosteum and intercostal muscle fascia. Care is taken to spare perforators during the elevation.
- During dissection, the pectoralis minor is encountered and preserved, allowing exposure of the thoracoacromial vessels. The lateral pectoral nerve and vessels are identified and divided if necessary to mobilize the flap fully.
- The thoracoacromial vessels serve as the primary pedicle (Figure 6.16). Dissection continues until adequate pedicle length is achieved for

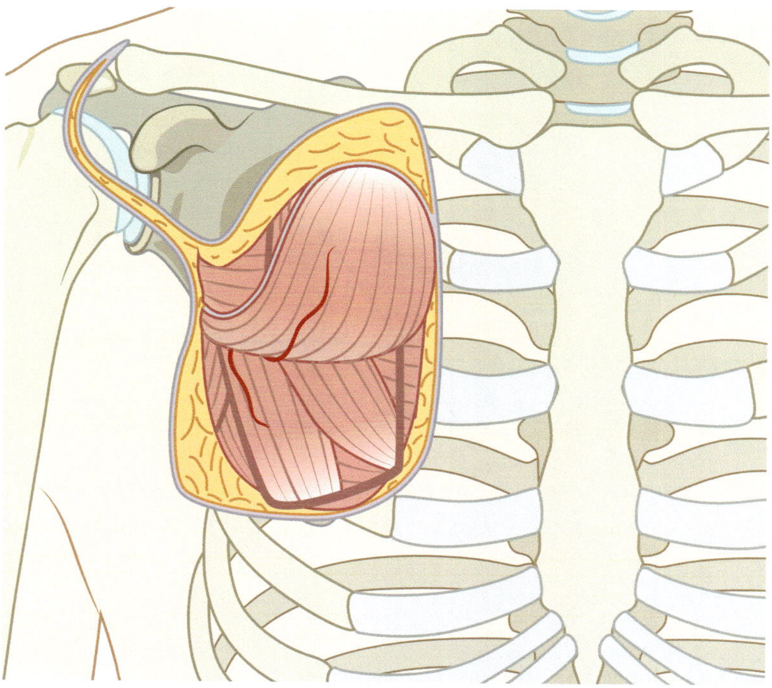

FIGURE 6.16 Vascular pedicle identified.

flap transposition. A tunnel is created above the clavicle and into the neck by dissecting subcutaneous tissue. The flap is gently pulled through this tunnel into the defect site, ensuring no tension on the pedicle.

- The flap is inset with careful alignment to avoid tension, which can compromise vascular flow. Muscle, subcutaneous tissue, and skin layers are secured in layers. Adjustments are made to ensure the flap lies naturally without compromising blood supply.
- The donor site is closed primarily or with minimal undermining to achieve tension-free closure. In females, the sub-mammary incision offers a superior cosmetic outcome. Suction drains are placed to prevent seroma formation.
- Monitoring for vascular compromise through flap color and capillary refill is performed twice daily.
- Drains are maintained to reduce seroma formation.
- Standard wound care and precautions to prevent complications like flap necrosis or infection are followed.

Advantages

- **Reliable Blood Supply**: The thoracoacromial artery ensures robust vascularization, reducing the risk of flap ischemia.
- **Ease of Harvest**: The flap can be harvested without complex microvascular techniques, making it suitable for a wide range of settings.
- **Versatility**: The flap can address diverse reconstructive needs in the head, neck, and thoracic regions.
- **Minimal Donor Site Morbidity**: Aesthetic and functional outcomes are favorable, especially when the donor site is closed primarily.

Potential Complications

While the PMF is reliable, complications may include:

- Partial or complete flap necrosis due to vascular compromise.
- Shoulder weakness or limited mobility, especially with extensive muscle harvest.

- Infection or seroma at the donor or recipient site.
- Cosmetic concerns related to chest wall contour.

Conclusion

The PMF remains a cornerstone of reconstructive surgery for head, neck, and thoracic defects. Its straightforward harvest technique, predictable outcomes, and adaptability make it an indispensable tool in the reconstructive surgeon's repertoire.

THE NASOLABIAL FLAP

The nasolabial flap (NF) is a time-tested, versatile option for reconstructing small to moderate defects in the oral cavity. This flap utilizes the skin and subcutaneous tissue of the nasolabial fold, providing well-vascularized tissue with minimal donor site morbidity.

Anatomy

The NF is based on the tissue within the nasolabial fold, a natural crease that extends from the side of the nose to the corner of the mouth. The flap can be designed as either superiorly or inferiorly based, depending on the location of the defect. The blood supply is robust, primarily deriving from branches of the facial artery, specifically the angular artery for superiorly based flaps and the inferior labial artery for inferiorly based flaps. However, most cases are random patterns based on the rich subdermal plexus (Figure 6.17).

The flap consists of skin, subcutaneous tissue, and sometimes muscle, allowing for flexibility in addressing various defect requirements. The proximity to the oral cavity makes it an excellent local flap option, reducing the need for distant tissue transfer or microvascular techniques.

Indications for Use

The NF is indicated for reconstructing small to moderate defects in the oral cavity, particularly in the following scenarios:

- **Defects of the Oral Mucosa**: Reconstruction of defects in the floor of the mouth, buccal mucosa, lip, and alveolar ridge.
- **Patients with Comorbidities**: Ideal for patients who are not candidates for lengthy procedures or microvascular reconstruction.
- **Adjunct to Other Flaps**: Can be used in combination with other flaps to address complex defects.

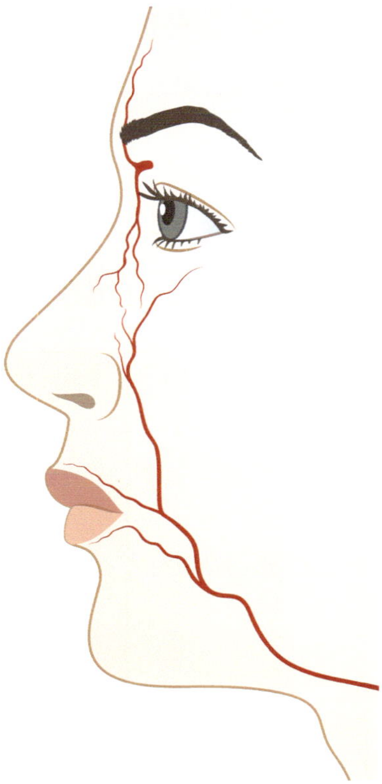

FIGURE 6.17 Anatomy of a nasolabial flap.

Procedure Overview

- **Marking the Flap**: Outline the flap within the nasolabial fold, ensuring adequate dimensions to cover the defect.
- **Dissection**: Elevate the flap carefully to preserve the vascular pedicle. For superiorly based flaps, preserve the angular artery; for inferiorly based flaps, preserve the inferior labial artery.
- **Transfer to Defect**: Create a tunnel or make an incision to transpose the flap into the oral cavity defect without tension.
- **Insetting the Flap**: Suture the flap into the defect, ensuring proper alignment and closure.
- **Donor Site Closure**: Close the donor site primarily, often resulting in minimal scarring due to the natural crease.

- **Flap Monitoring**: Regular assessment for signs of vascular compromise or infection.
- **Oral Hygiene**: Maintain cleanliness of the oral cavity to prevent infection.

Advantages

- **Simplicity**: The procedure is straightforward and can be performed under local anesthesia.
- **Proximity**: Close to the oral cavity, reducing operative time and complexity.
- **Good Blood Supply**: High flap survival rates due to robust vascularity.
- **Minimal Donor Site Morbidity**: Donor site scars are concealed within the nasolabial fold.

Potential Complications

- **Hair-Bearing Skin**: In male patients, the flap may introduce hair into the oral cavity.
- **Limited Reach**: May not adequately reach posterior defects without tension.
- **Potential for Facial Asymmetry**: Bilateral NLF reduce asymmetry.

Overuse can lead to noticeable differences in facial contour. Unsuitable for dentate patients with floor of the mouth defects.

- **Flap Necrosis**: Rare but may occur if the vascular pedicle is compromised.
- **Infection**: Preventable with proper hygiene and may require antibiotics if it occurs.
- **Salivary Fistula**: Uncommon but can develop if there is breakdown at the suture line.
- **Donor Site Scarring**: Usually minimal but may require revision in some cases.

Conclusion

The NF is a reliable and versatile option for reconstructing small to moderate oral cavity defects following cancer resection. Its simplicity, robust blood supply, and minimal donor site morbidity make it an attractive choice, especially for patients who may not be ideal candidates for more complex reconstructions. Careful patient selection, meticulous surgical technique, and diligent post-operative care are essential for optimal outcomes.

BUCCAL FAT PAD (BFP)

The BFP is a versatile and well-vascularized structure that can be used for reconstructing defects in the oral cavity and surrounding areas. Initially popularized for its use in closing oro-antral fistulas, the BFP has expanded its role in head and neck reconstruction due to its ease of harvest, excellent vascularity, and minimal morbidity. It is especially useful for smaller- to moderate-sized defects in the oral cavity, particularly after oncologic resections or trauma.

Anatomy

The BFP is a deep fat mass located between the buccinator muscle and other facial muscles like the masseter and zygomaticus major. It consists of several lobes that extend into the masticatory space, providing volume and cushioning in the cheek area. The fat pad is highly vascularized, primarily by branches of the maxillary artery, making it an ideal tissue for reconstructive purposes (Figure 6.18).

The average size of the BFP is about 9.6 cm^3, which is generally sufficient to cover moderate intra-oral defects. Its flexibility and proximity to the oral cavity make it a prime candidate for reconstructing various defects, especially within the mouth.

Indications for Use

The BFP is frequently used in the reconstruction of oral and maxillofacial defects, particularly when soft tissue coverage is required. Common indications include:

- **Oroantral Fistula Closure**: Often used following maxillary tooth extractions that have resulted in communication between the oral cavity and the maxillary sinus.

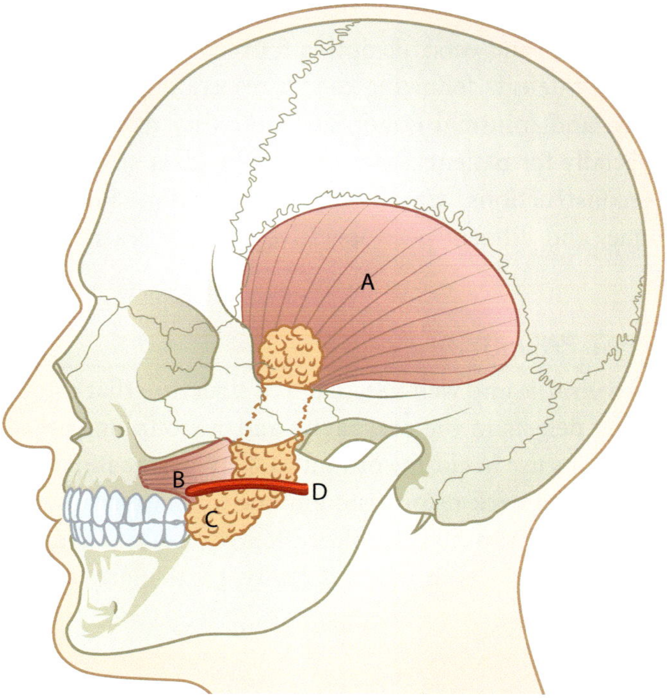

FIGURE 6.18 Anatomy of a buccal fat pad. A: Temporalis muscle, B: Buccinator muscle, C: Buccal fat pad, and D: Stensen's duct.

- **Palatal Defects**: For reconstruction after resection of oral tumors, congenital deformities, or trauma.
- **Buccal Mucosa Defects**: Following oncologic resection.
- **Floor of the Mouth and Alveolar Ridge Defects**: Where soft tissue volume is needed.

Procedure Overview

- The BFP is exposed through a small incision in the buccal mucosa, typically just posterior to the maxillary molars. A blunt dissection is performed through the mucosa and buccinator muscle, allowing the fat pad to be gently teased out of its fascial envelope. Care is taken to avoid damaging the fat pad's vascular pedicle to ensure its viability.
- Once the fat pad is exposed, it is carefully mobilized and drawn into the defect site. Gentle pressure externally to the cheek, anterior to the masseter muscle, to encourage controlled fat herniation.

- The flap can be rotated or advanced to fill defects in the palate, buccal mucosa, or other intra-oral regions. Due to the elasticity of the fat pad, it can be extended without tension to reach most parts of the oral cavity.
- After mobilizing the BFP into the defect, it is carefully sutured into place using absorbable sutures. The donor site, which is typically in the buccal mucosa, is either closed primarily or left to heal by secondary intention, depending on the size of the incision.

Advantages

The BFP offers numerous advantages in head and neck reconstruction:

- **Easy Accessibility**: The BFP is easily accessible through the oral cavity, eliminating the need for external incisions.
- **Minimal Morbidity**: Harvesting the fat pad causes little to no functional or aesthetic damage, with donor site morbidity being rare.
- **Excellent Vascularity**: The rich blood supply of the BFP ensures good integration into the defect and reduces the risk of necrosis.
- **Versatility**: The fat pad can be used to cover defects in various parts of the oral cavity, including the palate, buccal mucosa, and alveolar ridge.
- **Good Aesthetic Outcome**: The donor site inside the cheek is not visible externally, making it cosmetically appealing for patients.

Potential Complications

While the BFP is a reliable flap, complications can occur. Some of the potential issues include:

- **Partial Flap Necrosis**: If the vascular supply is compromised during harvest, the fat pad may undergo partial necrosis. Careful handling of the pedicle reduces this risk.
- **Volume Loss**: Some volume reduction occurs naturally as the fat pad integrates into the defect. However, this is generally not problematic for most reconstructions.
- **Donor Site Morbidity**: While rare, some patients may experience discomfort, infection, or scarring at the donor site.

- **Infection**: Proper post-operative care, including good oral hygiene and possibly antibiotics, can mitigate the risk of infection.
- **Mucosal Dehiscence**: If the flap is not properly secured or the patient does not follow post-operative care instructions, mucosal dehiscence may occur, requiring revision surgery.

Conclusion

The BFP is an excellent option for reconstructing soft tissue defects in the oral cavity. Its accessibility, robust blood supply, and versatility make it a preferred choice for surgeons dealing with moderate-sized defects. With proper surgical technique and post-operative care, the BFP provides reliable and aesthetically favorable outcomes with minimal donor site morbidity. Its use has become well established in head and neck reconstruction, offering a straightforward solution to complex defects.

PLATYSMA FLAP

The platysma flap is a reliable, thin, and versatile flap, ideal for reconstructing small to moderate soft tissue defects in the head and neck region. It is often used for intra-oral defects, lower facial reconstruction, and superficial skin coverage, especially when bulk is not required.

Candidates for the platysma flap are typically those with moderate, superficial defects that require thin, well-vascularized tissue for coverage. The platysma flap is often chosen in cases where free flap reconstruction may not be necessary or feasible. The flap can be used for both intra-oral and external defects, particularly in the lower face and neck.

Anatomy

The platysma muscle lies just under the skin of the neck, and the flap is harvested along with the overlying skin or as a muscle-only flap, depending on the defect. A Doppler ultrasound may be used to assess the vascular supply of the flap, primarily provided by the submental artery and transverse cervical artery.

Procedure Overview

- The skin paddle can be designed over the platysma muscle, typically 8–10 cm long and 3–5 cm wide, depending on the defect size. The flap can also be harvested as a muscle-only flap if no external coverage is required. The muscle is mobilized, preserving the blood supply and ensuring adequate reach for the defect (Figure 6.19).

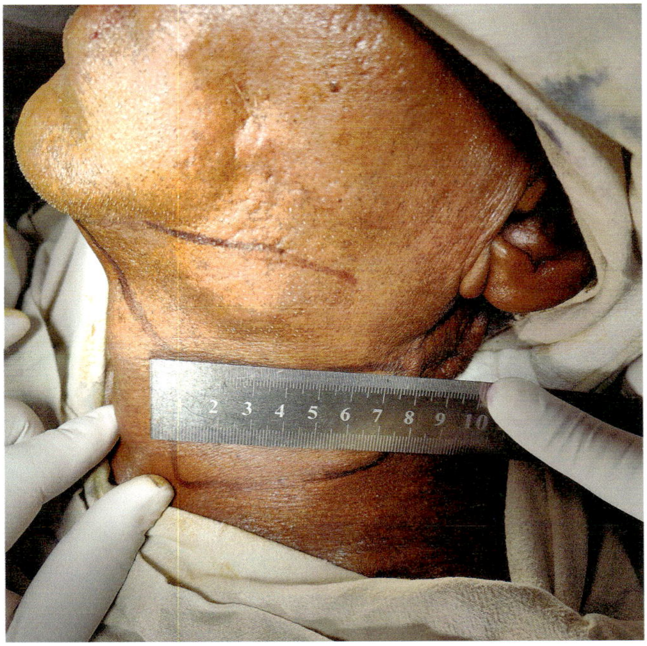

FIGURE 6.19 Skin markings.

- A horizontal incision is made in the lower neck, approximately 2.5 cm below the lower border of the mandible to preserve the marginal mandibular nerve. The incision begins at the lower border and extends along the anterior and posterior borders up to the subplatysmal layer. The skin over the platysma muscle is elevated carefully, preserving the blood supply.
- The platysma muscle is dissected free from the overlying skin and the underlying tissues. The muscle itself is thin, providing excellent pliability for reconstruction, and is preserved along with its blood supply from either the submental or transverse cervical artery (Figure 6.20).
- The width and length of the muscle flap are determined based on the defect being reconstructed. Then the incision at the superior margin is made down to the muscle only, taking care not to damage the muscle. This layer is raised up to or sometimes above the lower border of the mandible. The platysma is then carefully raised first at the posterior aspect up to the posterior belly of the digastric muscle, where the facial artery emerges superiorly

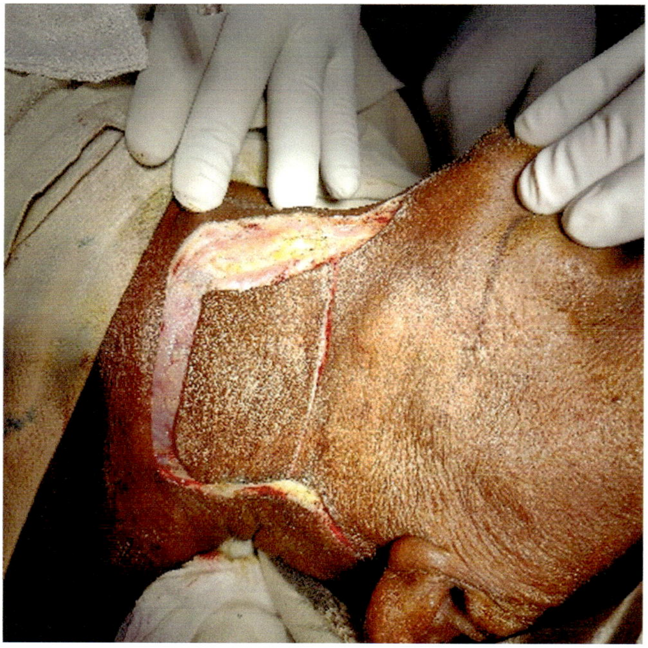

FIGURE 6.20 Flap raised.

- The vascular pedicle (submental) is identified and preserved throughout the flap harvesting process. Care must be taken to ensure the pedicle remains intact to maintain the flap's viability. The submental artery, arising from the facial artery at the inner surface of the mandible, can be very easily identified and preserved if extra care is taken at the antero-inferior border of the masseter muscle where the facial artery hooks around the lower border of the mandible.
- The flap is then raised up to the lower border of the mandible. Although the primary blood supply to the flap is the ipsilateral submental artery, it also receives supply from the ipsilateral mental, labial, and lingual arteries, as well as contralateral lingual and labial arteries.
- The flap is transposed to the defect through a subcutaneous tunnel or directly through an open incision, depending on the location of the defect. For intra-oral defects, the flap can be tunneled under the jaw and inset into the defect, while for external defects, it is positioned on the surface to provide skin coverage.

- The platysma flap is carefully sutured into the defect, ensuring that there is no tension on the flap or pedicle. For through-and-through defects, the platysma flap can be folded to provide both internal and external coverage.
- The donor site is typically closed primarily, especially if a skin paddle is not harvested. Drains are placed to avoid hematoma or seroma formation, particularly in cases where a large skin paddle is harvested. The scar is often well-hidden within the natural creases of the neck.

Advantages

- Thin and pliable, ideal for superficial or small intra-oral defects.
- Excellent for lower facial and neck reconstruction, with minimal donor site morbidity.
- Reliable vascularity when based on the submental or transverse cervical artery.
- Can be harvested with or without a skin paddle, making it versatile for various types of defects.
- Suitable for one-stage reconstruction.
- *Aesthetic Outcomes*: The flap's thin nature and the hidden scar in the neck crease often result in excellent aesthetic outcomes, especially for external facial defects.

Potential Complications

- The flap provides minimal bulk, which may not be suitable for large or deep defects.
- Care must be taken to avoid tension on the flap, particularly when tunneling it for intra-oral defects.
- Flap viability is highly dependent on preserving the vascular pedicle, and the surgeon must be cautious during dissection.
- Limited reach to the upper face or scalp due to the size of the flap and the vascular pedicle.
- *Vascular Considerations*: Careful attention must be paid to the vascular supply, particularly when harvesting the flap from the submental artery. Any damage to these vessels can compromise flap viability.

Conclusion

The platysma flap is a reliable, thin, and versatile flap, ideal for reconstructing small to moderate soft tissue defects in the head and neck region.

INFRAHYOID FLAP (IHF)

The IHF is a robust and versatile reconstructive option for moderate-sized defects in the head and neck region, particularly the floor of the mouth and lower alveolus. The flap is based on the superior thyroid artery and is well-suited for reconstructing intra-oral and facial defects where a reliable tissue with good bulk is needed.

Anatomy

The IHF primarily involves the strap muscles, including the sternohyoid, sternothyroid, and omohyoid (which is sometimes partially included).

The flap's vascularization is derived from the superior thyroid artery, a branch of the external carotid artery. Additional contributions may come from the inferior thyroid artery, ensuring robust blood supply. Venous drainage occurs through veins that accompany the arteries and eventually drain into the internal jugular vein.

Procedure Overview

- The vascular supply of the flap, predominantly the superior thyroid artery, is assessed using Doppler ultrasound if necessary.
- The IHF is harvested as a myocutaneous flap after ipsilateral modified radical or selective neck dissection is completed. Technically, the harvest of the IHF does not interfere with the extent of the neck dissection, since this flap lies in the central compartment of the neck, medial to the carotid artery at neck level VI.
- A careful pinch test can determine the skin's laxity and how much tissue can be harvested. The dimensions of the skin paddle are tailored based on the defect size and tissue requirements (Figure 6.21).
- A curvilinear incision is made at the level of the hyoid bone, extending laterally across the neck to provide access to the infrahyoid muscles. The incision allows for a skin paddle to be harvested based on the required dimensions.

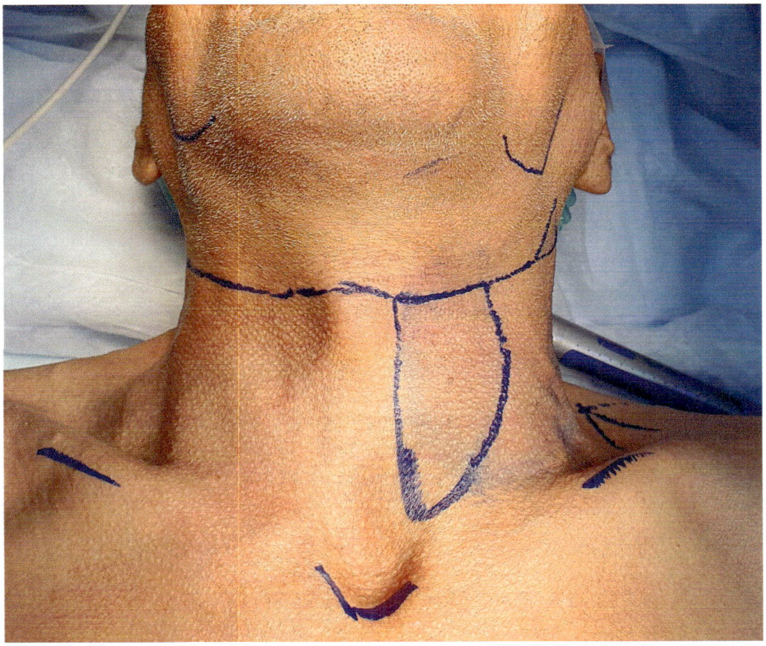

FIGURE 6.21 Skin markings for an infrahyoid flap.

- The skin, platysma, and subcutaneous tissues are elevated to expose the infrahyoid muscles, which include the sternohyoid, sternothyroid, omohyoid, and thyrohyoid muscles. The superior thyroid artery and the associated veins are carefully dissected and preserved to maintain the flap's vascular supply.
- The skin paddle is tailored based on the defect. A 6–8 cm long and 3–4 cm wide skin paddle is typical, but this can vary depending on the size of the defect. The muscle is detached at its lower attachment, preserving the superior vascular pedicle.
- The flap is carefully raised, preserving its vascular pedicle and the superior thyroid artery. The flap's mobility is assessed to ensure it can reach the defect without tension.
- After harvesting, the flap is transposed to the defect through a subcutaneous tunnel or a neck incision. It can be used to reconstruct defects of the oral cavity, lower lip, floor of the mouth, or lower alveolus. In cases of through-and-through defects, the flap can be folded to provide both internal and external coverage.

- The donor site is closed primarily if possible. Drains are often placed to prevent seroma or hematoma formation. The donor site scar is generally well-concealed in the neck crease, making it aesthetically acceptable.

Advantages

- Provides reliable bulk for moderate-sized defects.
- Good vascularity due to the superior thyroid artery.
- Can be harvested with minimal morbidity.
- A single-stage procedure with a relatively easy technique.
- Suitable for a variety of head and neck reconstructions.

Potential Complications

- Flap bulk may be excessive in small defects.
- The donor site may require careful closure, especially in patients with limited skin laxity.
- The vascular pedicle must be handled carefully to avoid complications with the flap's perfusion.
- Pre-operative evaluation of the superior thyroid artery and vein's anatomy is crucial to avoid intra-operative complications.

Conclusion

The IHF provides an excellent option for reconstruction of moderate-sized defects, particularly in patients with floor of the mouth or lower alveolus defects.

While the flap provides ample bulk, careful thinning may be necessary to avoid excessive tissue in smaller defects. Care must be taken when using the flap in patients with metastatic or recurrent disease.

Index

Note: Locators in *italics* represent figures in the text.

G

H

I

J

K

L

R

W

Z

For Product Safety Concerns and Information please contact our EU representative GPSR@taylorandfrancis.com Taylor & Francis Verlag GmbH, Kaufingerstraße 24, 80331 München, Germany